THE LIFE WELL LIVED

www.**transworldireland**.ie

www.**penguin**.co.uk

Also by Professor Jim Lucey

Understanding Psychiatric Treatment
(co-edited with Dr G. O'Mahony)

In My Room

THE LIFE WELL LIVED

The Therapeutic Journey to Recovery and Wellbeing

Professor Jim Lucey

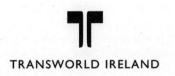

TRANSWORLD IRELAND

TRANSWORLD IRELAND PUBLISHERS
Penguin Random House Ireland, Morrison Chambers, 32 Nassau Street, Dublin 2, Ireland
www.transworldireland.ie

Transworld Ireland is part of the Penguin Random House group of companies
whose addresses can be found at global.penguinrandomhouse.com

Penguin
Random House
UK

First published in the UK and Ireland in 2017
by Transworld Ireland
an imprint of Transworld Publishers

A CIP catalogue record for this book
is available from the British Library.

ISBN 9781848272330

Typeset in 12/14.5pt Minion Pro by Falcon Oast Graphic Art Ltd.
Printed and bound by Clays Ltd, Bungay, Suffolk.

Penguin Random House is committed to a sustainable
future for our business, our readers and our planet. This book
is made from Forest Stewardship Council® certified paper.

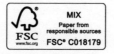

1 3 5 7 9 10 8 6 4 2

Note to Readers

As with all books, this one contains the opinions and ideas of the author. It is
intended to provide helpful and informative material on the subjects addressed
and is sold with the understanding that the author and publisher are not engaged
in rendering medical, health, psychological or any other kind of personal
professional services or therapy in the book. The reader should consult his or her
medical, health, psychological or other competent professional before adopting
any of the concepts in this book or drawing inferences from it. The content of this
book, by its very nature, is general, whereas each reader's situation is unique.
Therefore, as with all books of this nature, the purpose is to provide general
information rather than address individual situations, which books by their very
nature cannot do.

The author and publisher specifically disclaim all responsibility for any liability,
loss, or risk, personal or otherwise, which is incurred as a consequence, directly or
indirectly, of the use and application of any of the contents of this book.

In Memory of Professor Aidan Halligan.

'It's about doing the right thing on a difficult day.'

Come to the edge.
We might fall.
Come to the edge.
It's too high!
COME TO THE EDGE!
And they came,
And he pushed,
And they flew.

Christopher Logue

Contents

Foreword

It is well recognized that one in four adults in their lifetime will develop a psychiatric disorder. Thus every family in the land will be affected directly or indirectly by the issues of mental health. It is also well established that 50 per cent of mental illnesses in adulthood originate before the age of fifteen, and three-quarters start before the age of twenty-four. The task for mental health professionals and policy-makers is clear; it is the prevention of psychiatric disorders and mental health promotion.

Mental health and wellbeing are beginning to receive the serious attention they deserve. Mental wellbeing is about the ability to form relationships, function effectively in various arenas, and lead a life that is full of hope and aspiration. Resilience and wellbeing go hand in hand. Resilience is about the capacity to manage stress no matter its source, and to bounce back after distress – and the ability to do so repeatedly.

We all know people who are not fazed by any type or level of stress, whereas others tend to give in and respond in a more passive way. Of course individual responses are very strongly influenced by cultural factors and by the patterns of child-rearing. As we are beginning to learn more about what happens in attachment patterns and childhood, we are able to understand patterns of response in adulthood. Mental illness carries a larger burden in comparison with physical illnesses such as cancer and heart disease, yet discrimination and stigma against mental illness are rife. One of the reasons that may well contribute to stigma is self-stigma in mental health professionals, indicating that somehow professionals are ashamed of what we deal with on a daily basis

– our inability to convince policy-makers and the public that we do a very good job under very difficult conditions, dealing with complex sets of symptoms, models of explanation and those of care. We need to take pride in what we do and this volume offers a significant way forward.

Another complicating factor is the artificial Cartesian dichotomy between mind and body. Although Descartes may not have meant such rigid divisions, in western psychiatry this has become often very difficult to navigate. The common isolation of psychiatric hospitals and asylums created an era of mystique about what we do and how we treat our patients, and this isolation may well have further contributed to being stigmatized.

In an easy to read and follow description of recovery and wellbeing Professor Jim Lucey has demonstrated a way of communicating with patients, their carers, families and members of the public. He sets his stall by defining what is understood by wellbeing, resilience and stigma, and what diagnosis means. Furthermore, he differentiates clearly between types of treatment and therapy. Illustrated by poignant narratives and reports from sessions, these are as much about a patient's progress as they are about Professor Lucey's learning, development and growth. There is no doubt that access, availability and affordability of therapies are at the heart of any service planning, development and delivery, no matter which part of the world patients and their psychiatrists live in. The choice of treatments depends upon what the patient's needs are and what is available locally, and how with care the need and treatment are mapped. Mental illness needs to be understood as a mixture of biopsychosocial factors, and therefore therapeutic interventions have to be looked at in the same context, even if one or more of the three options are given preference. Spiritual interventions may also help in some settings. The choice of various therapies is strongly influenced by available human resources, but also training and supervisory opportunities. Professor Lucey quite rightly reminds us that this approach must be seen in the context of a human-rights framework. He argues that ideally interventions will look at the needs rather than simply focusing on management of diagnoses. By helping, enabling and empowering our patients, we can ensure that they recover and function to the best of their abilities. In engaging patients, the best option is to get individual patients to see what may be relevant and meaningful for them. Helping them to develop more mindful recovery means that patients are encouraged to develop restorative capacities such as acceptance, commitment, courage, compassion and kindness. Any engagement with the process of therapy can empower recovery. A major part of this learning must rely on education and this is what Professor Lucey has done in this slim volume.

Just because this volume is easy to read does not make it simple. It is a tribute to Professor Lucey's style that he can convey complex ideas in an easy to understand manner. There are many reasons why this book is important. The foremost is about education and the de-stigmatization of mental illness and people with mental illness. In a careful communication, this volume offers lots to learn.

Dinesh Bhugra CBE
Emeritus Professor of Mental Health and
Cultural Diversity, King's College, London;
President, World Psychiatric Association
May 2017

Introduction

MENTAL HEALTH IS OUR most valuable possession. We may not see it as priceless or fundamental, but actually everything we care about is critically dependent on it: our ability to live, to work and to love.

With this book, I hope to introduce to you five therapeutic paths to wellness. Each is based on genuine experience of modern mental healthcare and they are all supported by respected research and study. Mental health is intangible. It's difficult to speak of it without adding to misunderstanding. Likewise mental healthcare can be complex. My hope is to illustrate in a straightforward fashion the practical ways in which these talking and listening therapies work effectively in the modern era. Of course, this therapy route may not be for everybody, and I fully respect this. Equally, it is important to remember that therapy could be something life changing and truly special.

Many different factors contribute to an effective therapy but two key elements are essential. The first is engagement, the second is continuity. Engagement with therapy requires a degree of determination. The result is a relationship between the therapist and the individual seeking recovery. We call this 'the therapeutic relationship' and it is precious. Its continuity depends on kindness at all times and perseverance for those times when things do not appear to go to plan or when the road ahead seems long and difficult.

In my view, these modern treatments illustrate a progression in therapy that is hopeful, humane and uplifting. My ultimate intention, my real aim, is to bring more attention to the potential for progress in mental healthcare and so, by illustrating some of its newer treatments, to shine a positive light into the psycho-therapeutic world, which is so often feared and misunderstood.

Even still, my own personal witness and that of my colleagues would not be enough to validate these treatments. An objective evidence base is essential and for this reason I have not included therapies unless they are supported by published objective evidence. By this I mean something more than a description of a theory or an outline of an ideological position. Granted, the development of any new treatment has to start from somewhere and theory is a good place to start, but the proof of the pudding must be in the eating. Modern therapy has to be seen to work.

Those paths I have included have this objective evidence of effectiveness – although I acknowledge that standards of this evidence do vary. By 'evidence base' I simply mean that each of these therapies is supported by substantial peer-reviewed pub-lished research addressing the important questions about when and where and for whom the therapy is effective.

My experience, and the work I have undertaken with colleagues in our multidisciplinary teams, has shown me that these therapies can help to restore wellbeing in men and women in great distress. These restorative benefits have become even more apparent as time has gone by and so my personal witness of recovery has compelled me to write more about them.

This book is divided into two parts. The first part sets out some general principles about what it is to be well and how therapy can help to achieve recovery. The second part is made up of a number of case studies which hopefully will illustrate the therapeutic process as it is put into action.

My hope is that these personal histories will reveal an emer-ging arc of recovery achieved through developments in cognitive behavioural therapy. These have been informed by concepts such as mindfulness, compassion and acceptance that have helped to connect these therapies to real-life recovery. Modern cognitive behavioural therapies promote new skills and new feelings, leading to renewed growth and wellbeing. This recovery requires hope and imagination. Throughout the book we will revisit some of these concepts so as to illustrate what is meant by them. To do this more vividly I have chosen to illustrate these therapies in narrative form – specifically in dialogue – so that they will come to being as stories about real therapy and real life. For whatever the specifics of therapy may be, the real change practitioners are the people themselves.

We will meet seven individuals in this book – Tara, Laura, Robert, Barbara, Arthur, Patricia and Joseph. Through each of them, we will see different changes in behaviour and thinking. And hopefully we will see more still – since these are somewhat limited parameters for the life well lived. What this book will actually show us is how these people return again and again to their journeys and how ultimately each person creates their own path to wellness.

I believe it is time to talk more about the actual process and practice of modern cognitive behavioural psychotherapy. I hope to encourage more of us to talk about our mental health treatment and about our journey to wellness. By attempting to show what actually unfolds in therapy, I hope to encourage a more authentic conversation about mental healthcare. My belief is that this openness will enable many more of us to ask important questions about our mental health and wellness. Asking these questions could be the beginning of another recovery. And that is what promoting wellness is all about.

This is a very personal view about the modern era of psycho-therapy – it is not a practice manual or a substitute for training. At one level, these are simply stories about real-life experiences. So please consider this book an invitation from me to you, to dis-cover how someone's path to recovery may be enhanced by engagement with modern mental healthcare. Maybe by listening to these therapeutic journeys we can learn something about each other and about how a recovery can be achieved.

Jim Lucey

PART I

1

What Does It Mean to Be Well?

IF YOU HAVE EVER lost your mental health, even temporarily, then you will already know about the special relationship that exists between mental wellness and every other aspect of your life. On the other hand, if you have never experienced a mental health issue the subject of mental disorder might seem like a distant concept. So why should you be concerned about mental health now?

The reality is this. The chances are high that any one of us will have a mental health problem at some stage in our life. The figures are striking. In fact, one in six of us will have a mental health problem in the next twelve months. And when this happens, mental health will suddenly become a very personal issue. The same risk applies to those we care most about in the world. Whether we know it or not, someone we love, some family member or friend, is in mental distress at this very moment. This distress is happening right now, even if we never speak about it.

Of course, it could be that you already know a great deal about your mental health and about how it is lost and found. It could be that you have already rebuilt your health based on the deepest personal experience of mental distress. The insights gained through a recovery are invaluable. When we share these accounts of our journey to health, we realize that the lessons we have learned are not unique. There is a universal wisdom gleaned by human beings who have experienced mental distress and have come back to fully enjoy everyday life once again. This wisdom leads us to understand what it means to be well.

What Is Wellness?

We live in a time when the attributes of wellness are constantly being redefined. In the past, many people in my profession spent decades trying to describe what it means to be unwell, without necessarily understanding what it means to be well. Now much of that focus on illness has changed and so a vast body of research has emerged, within psychology and elsewhere, examining the features of wellness.

The findings are remarkably consistent. Most people agree that the past emphasis on questions of pathology has been relatively unproductive. In recent times, much more has been learned by those researchers and thinkers who are asking more open and universal questions: What are the common characteristics of positive mental health? What is wellbeing? How can more of us be well and how can we stay well?

At its simplest level 'wellness' can be seen as a state of being in good physical and mental health. Unfortunately, although it's a start, this definition tells us very little. We need a broader, more nuanced definition of what it is to be well in order to understand wellness in human terms. A more informative definition of wellness (or what we might call the life well lived) should include many dimensions of lived experience. One such inclusive definition of human wellness describes eight dimensions of wellness.[1]

These have been promoted by many agencies, most prominently in the USA by the Substance Abuse and Mental Health Services Administration (SAMHSA). So what are these eight dimensions of wellness?[2]

[1] M. Swarbrick, 'A Wellness Approach', *Psychiatric Rehabilitation Journal*, Vol. 29(4), 2006, pp. 311–14.

[2] The eight dimensions can be viewed at www.samhsa.gov/wellness-initiative/eight-dimensions-wellness, where much of their health promotion data is also available.

- Emotional
- Environmental
- Financial
- Intellectual
- Occupational
- Physical
- Social
- Spiritual

It's an impressive list. To my mind, none of these dimensions could or should be omitted by any meaningful description of wellness, but wellness by this definition will not be easily achieved. Surely it would be a tall order to succeed in all of these areas all of the time. Do we need to excel in every one of these arenas in order to live well? This may be a great list, but in reality few of us triumph in many of these dimensions even some of the time! Any definition of wellness needs to be broad enough to show how multifaceted and human the well-lived life could be, but in my view a more forgiving, practical approach is required.

Perhaps we could learn about wellness by observing those who have good health. This was the basic approach of one remarkable group of scientists who questioned the meaning of wellness. Curiously these were not a group of clinical scientists but a group of economists, environmentalists and development campaigners who call themselves the New Economics Foundation (NEF). Rather than describe wellness in an aspirational sense they looked to describe the tangible characteristics of people who already see themselves as 'well'. So, what can we learn about wellness by studying the well?

It's worth pondering for a moment why this question was of interest to a group of economists and environmentalists. In fact, the answer is simple. They understood the economic value of mental health to society. Our collective mental health is societal wealth. When the NEF looked back at the global financial collapse of 2008, and the human consequences of this and other economic disasters, they understood the need for an objective examination of the wider economy, including the mental health of the whole

9

population. The economic solutions for any nation are about more than restoration of growth or management of the money supply. Free markets are about people, so an economic recovery depends on a human recovery. This is why the analysis of mental wellness produced by the economists of the NEF is so relevant.

Of course not everyone agrees with this. Some people still see wellness as the inevitable privilege of the rich. But is wellness only for the well-off? Or is it possible to consider wellness in a different way, so that we hope for a society which is *well* for everyone and not just *well-off* for some? To answer these questions, it is necessary to unpick the complex relationship between our economic well-being and our mental wellbeing.

In my experience, the mental health of society is clearly inter-twined with its economic wellbeing, but this relationship is not linear. Illness (and not just mental illness) does correlate with poverty, but the same is not true for wealth and happiness. Increasing happiness is not exclusively connected to greater wealth. When NEF reviewed the data, they combined their find-ings into an analysis known as meta-analysis, looking at all the published factors associated with mental wellness. They concluded that five characteristics were typical of people who are mentally well. Arising from these five factors, the NEF created a project entitled 'Five Ways to Wellbeing'.[3]

These five ways describe the characteristics of people whose mental health is robust. We can think of the five ways as a sort of mental health exercise. It's behaviourism at a population level. The proposition is that if we were able to do these things, we too could be mentally well. So, what are these five ways to wellness?

- Connect
- Be Active
- Take Notice

___
[3] These findings are available as a PDF and they can be seen at ww. neweconomics.org/projects/entry/five-ways-to-wellbeing.

- Keep Learning
- Give

So, let us ask this mental health question. Do these attributes describe life lived well? Is NEF right? Are these the characteristics of the mentally healthy? Well, let's see.

Certainly, the first two – being in communication with others and being active each day – are bound to be good for you. We human beings are, after all, social animals. This engagement and activity is the antithesis of the isolation and immobility which is so common with those who are distressed. Likewise taking notice of each moment and savouring it for itself means living in the present and this is truly the essence of mindfulness. (We will consider mindfulness in more depth in Chapter 3.) A mindful experience of peace is not to be confused with a desire for escape. In reality it is by taking note of each moment that we become truly aware.

A willingness to keep learning is a mark of our adaptability and this is the hallmark of any successful life. It is also a hallmark of any successful species. And then lastly there is giving. There is so much to say about the value of giving, and not necessarily giving in a material sense: this is about giving our time, our energy and our mental space to share with others. It's also about giving to ourselves, giving time, giving ground, giving way and even giving up. There is so much wellness achieved by giving.

So there we have it. Surely now we know the stuff we all have to do to live life well. We know exactly what a well-lived life looks like and so we should know what it requires. What more is there to be said? Surely we should just get on with things – 'Just do it'. As things turn out, though, this is not one of the most helpful of slogans for the pursuit of wellness.

We may have the recipe for wellness, but it's not easy to follow it all of the time. Why is this? One reason is because of stress. You see, life – even a well-lived one – can be stressful.

The Life Well Lived and Stress

There is a relationship between our wellness and the stress in our life, but this relationship is a two-way street. To live well is to experience both good and bad things at the same time and yet to continue living even though we experience them throughout our life. Not all stress is bad for us, but we are all shaped by it for better or worse. There is the everyday rush for work or school, the pressure to achieve. And haven't we all loved and lost? Admittedly, some losses are greater than others and some leave indelible marks. Most of our stresses, however, are met with the resilience that is characteristic of human beings. Most people recover and so our expectation of recovery is not merely a dream. In my view, it is a basic human right.

Stress? What Stress?

We will all suffer from some stress; there is no getting past that reality in modern life. If we fail to acknowledge stress, we can be sure of one thing. Many negative things will happen to us. We will see some examples of this stress phenomenon later in the book when we meet a few of my patients, but for now it's sufficient to say one thing: any guidance on living life well that fails to acknowledge the universality of stress is, frankly, way off the mark.

Life for many is very stressful. And worse still, this stress is not evenly distributed. Stress is not fair. It comes plentifully to some and not so much to others. When it does visit us, it often comes when we least expect it – and its impact on each of us seems unique and unforeseen. Even though stress is universal, not all stress is the same. Life is much harder for some people than it is for others.

For example, stress comes in a stream of unrelenting tasks and practical struggles for many people; the daily grind of work or lack of work, and conflicts with others can combine to make any life a personal struggle. For others life stress is more sudden in onset and more sharply destructive. These traumas are also part of life stress and they are unavoidable.

Stress and suffering are universal experiences yet individual ones at the same time. This paradox is part of what it is to be human and social. At some stage we will all experience a degree of pain. We may rationalize this by saying 'where there is no pain, there is no gain'. We may even see such suffering as the basis for some of the personal victories that make our life meaningful and rewarding. But the truth is that so much suffering is without any potential gain. Mental suffering surely falls into this category. It is an especially frustrating form of painful experience. Sometimes all we can do is wait for it to pass. Mental suffering is not contagious, but its potential to descend upon any of us is an ever-present reality which seems to serve no purpose.

This may sound shocking to some. There are those who see value in every form of human experience, even painful ones. Some view melancholic grief, for example, as the price we must pay for loving someone that we have lost. But if this is true, then I would suggest that little is gained by paying such a price. It is true that mental suffering does pass and sometimes we must simply wait until it does, but is waiting in pain the price we must pay to regain a better life?

The experience of stress does pass, but it need not destroy our ability to live life well again. Actually our strength may be rebuilt in the context of much stress. We can learn even in an environment where we experience reversal, disappointment and loss. It is a mistake to see the longed-for life well lived as a stress-free, charmed existence enjoyed only by a lucky few. We can live well with stress.

So let us start by agreeing that being well does not mean that we will never feel stressed or tired or ill. Most of us will become ill but most of us will recover. Typically we can find a way to live well again, even though this sometimes involves a degree of continued stress and even pain. The life well lived may contain such pain, but as it continues it can also include joy and laughter, connection and love.

How can this be? There is one reason. We are human beings and this fact means that we have a remarkable capacity for resilience. (This is a topic we will look at in more depth later in this chapter – see What Is Resilience?, p. 24).

The connection between stress and wellness is an important and also a hopeful one. It is not the most pleasant place to start from, but stress may be the point from which we kickstart our journey back towards wellness. Indeed, it is only when we acknowledge that stress and wellness are linked in this way that we can start to view it as a sort of opportunity, a crossroads from which we can travel on, moving towards further distress or hopefully towards wellness.

Wellness vs Illness: A Matter of Choice?

Wellness is not a static or absolute state. It is possible to live life well and still have significant illness. There are degrees of wellness. It is on a continuum and so at any one time some are more well than others, but just because wellness is on a human spectrum does not mean it is a matter of individual choice. Experiencing illness or suffering is not a desirable option. Being depressed, for example, is not simply a bad lifestyle choice. Although men and women experiencing depression reproach themselves every day, the truth is that they did not make a choice to lead a miserable life. Recognizing this helps to resolve guilt and self-reproach, and this is an important step during the process of recovery. It involves more than choosing to avoid a set of unhealthy options to recover from depression, and remaining well involves something more than the decision to do or not to do any potentially toxic thing.

A healthy life is a balanced one. Restoration of our mental equilibrium coincides with the reintegration of our lives within ourselves and with the lives of others. In my experience recovery always involves some form of personal and social reconnection. This is illustrated frequently by my patients in Part II. But what makes this reconnection possible? There are many factors. There is no single recipe, but an essential ingredient is 'acceptance'. We will see some examples of this phenomenon later in this book, but for now it is sufficient to say that every successful voyage to recovery includes a good measure of acceptance. By this I mean acknowledgement of the whole of our human experience and also the recognition that our experience must include suffering and illness to some degree.

In this life, very few of us will survive without any illness. Actually many of us will have two or more enduring illnesses in our lifetime. Nowadays, we can expect to live long lives – hopefully living, loving and working despite our many enduring illnesses. If wellness were limited to those without illness, then the healthy among us would make up a very exclusive club indeed. If this were the case, very few of us could ever hope to say that we were very well for very long.

Thankfully, wellness is not something that is inevitably lost through illness. Wellness is something that can be discovered throughout life and even in the context of illness and suffering. And so this is another paradox about our health: being well can include the experience of being unwell. We can recover our wellness while also being unwell, to some degree.

Medicine vs Therapy: Which Way Is Best for Recovery?

In some ways, we live in blessed times. Nowadays, most of us will make a full recovery even after we experience mental distress. Even still, despite many advances, much more needs to be done. Since we now know that recovery is possible, why is it that so many people still wait – sometimes for years – for the assistance they need? Why is mental healthcare so often the proverbial tin can to be kicked down the road? What is it about our society that we deny mental health the priority it deserves, perhaps the greatest priority, even though this denial means our distress is amplified and so recovery becomes more difficult for everyone?

Part of the problem lies in the complexity of the mental healthcare system, which is historically filled with disputing professionals and differing ideological points of view. As a result even today, despite so much evidence of real effectiveness, it can be hard to plot a realistic route towards better mental health.

So imagine what it would be like if we could see a clear way forward to mental health, one that would allow each person to live his or her life to the full. Would we have a different attitude towards mental healthcare if we shared this evidence-based direction? Even though we know our resources vary a great deal, and not everyone has the same needs, imagine what it would be like if we could all agree to enhance our mental health using all the tools we have? But what are these mental healthcare tools? Do they involve medicine or therapy, or perhaps even both? To date, there has been too little agreement on this point. Mental health practitioners frequently dispute with each other about these seemingly unanswerable questions. There are many reasons for this conflict. Psychological medicine has often been seen as untrustworthy and excessively pharmacological – or, as one patient put it to me, 'heavy on medication and low on insight'. Psychotherapy and counselling are also easily parodied. Many patients who embark on a talking therapy express their concerns about this straight off. Some fear that it will be non-directive and unhelpful – 'just tea and sympathy' – a soft approach that is drawn out and ineffective. Others fear that therapy will be too directive, even punitive – an 'emotional boot camp'. Both extremes, in my experience, are travesties of the truth. Neither pole is helpful. Authentic mental healthcare is not about adopting absolute positions. Meaningful mental healthcare is holistic and humane, and its priority is the restoration of human wellbeing.

Stigma: Why Is It Still an Issue?

Every conversation with someone in distress is different, but sooner or later all our mental health talk comes back to one issue. This issue is stigma. It cannot be ignored. My patients tell me they have to face it every day and that is why it matters so much to them. Stigma defines their experience of mental health difficulty and it remains the biggest challenge in all of mental healthcare.

Perhaps if we could overcome stigma, this would be the greatest therapy of all. So, what is stigma?

To stigmatize someone is to alienate them, to exclude them or discriminate against them because they appear different or threatening in some way. Stigma is not a phenomenon unique to mental health. Around the world and for all of time people have been stigmatized because of their race, their colour, their gender, their sexual orientation and countless other so-called 'differences' from the main herd.

Labelling others through stigma allows one group to unite by marginalizing another. This works at many different levels to alienate: politically, socially and professionally. We have seen stigma used as a tool by those in power. This way others can be blamed for things we fear. Whatever its specifics, this much is true: stigma is always a negative experience for the individual who is stigmatized.

We are still quick to use it. Stigma allows us to sidestep difficult truths about people and events that we cannot easily understand. Take, for example, the rise in global terrorism. The causes of this phenomenon include many complex geopolitical and historical forces, and these are often hard to accept, to understand or control, but regardless of their real causes terrorist crimes are usually first described as acts of 'evil' or 'madness'. The effect is to obscure or at least delay a deeper consideration of a life's tragic history.

Stigma allows us to defend and even justify more negative aspects of ourselves, such as our capacity for malice or greed. In many societies, people with mental health difficulties feel alienated and alone as a result of the hostile responses to their mental distress and behaviours.

But stigma makes life much more challenging for those with mental health problems. For example, it is more difficult to get a mortgage or life assurance after a mental breakdown. It may also be harder to form a relationship with someone if you have ever had a diagnosis of mental illness. Imagine how difficult this must be, and you will see why my patients often feel the need to conceal their experience of illness. Stigma has the effect of driving mental health problems underground. My patients tell me that because of stigma they find it necessary to circumvent many practical day-to-day questions. After all, how do you tell your employer, your banker or your lover that you have had a mental breakdown? There are no good ways to handle these disclosures. Every day people seek answers to these questions, but there are no easy answers. So what do we do about stigma?

There are a number of common anti-stigma initiatives. One strategy is to challenge stigma by increasing public awareness about mental health and mental difficulty.[4] Another is to fight stigma by increasing personal advocacy for mental recovery.

Attempts to reduce stigma by increasing public understanding have had limited success. Obviously there is great merit in increasing public knowledge of healthy living, of a healthy diet and exercise, of the value of wellness overall, but despite these initiatives stigmatic attitudes towards people who experience mental health difficulty have been very resistant to change. In addition, information about biological and psychological causes of mental distress may not change stigmatic attitudes.[5] The real stigmatic issues involve the distrust of the population for those who experience mental health challenges. Mobilizing public awareness may be a first step, but what should the message be?

One problem is that mental health is not yet accepted as a common value based on universal human rights. Perhaps if access to mental healthcare was seen as a human right more people would engage with it and so stigmatic attitudes would also soften. A greater constituency might be built around mental health

[4] G. Sampogna, I. Bakolis, S. Evans-Lacko, E. Robinson, G. Thornicroft and C. Henderson, 'The impact of social marketing campaigns on reducing mental health stigma: Results from the 2009–2014 Time to Change programme', *European Psychiatry*, Vol. 16(40), Dec. 2016, pp. 116–22.

[5] A. E. Lyndon, A. Crowe, K. L. Wuensch, S. L. McCammon and K. B. Davies, 'College students' stigmatization of people with mental illness: familiarity, implicit person theory, and attribution', *Journal of Mental Health*, Vol. 25, Nov. 2016.

advocacy if we were to accept that mental health is an issue for us all. Mistrust of others might also diminish if we accepted we were all in this together. So far at least, public awareness campaigns have failed to build this sense of universal solidarity for those with mental difficulty.

Instead those with mental health problems commonly feel excluded and ashamed of their difficulties and this shame is sometimes called 'self-stigma'. It is one of the most destructive forms of stigmatic experience. Shame persists even though some attitudes to mental health are changing. After all, more people are willing to acknowledge their anxiety and depression, and more people are likely to talk openly about these issues than ever before. Much of this progressive shift has been put down to the work of popular celebrities, who have spoken freely about their mental health difficulties. By being open about their panic attacks, anxiety, addictions or depression, these individuals do a great service. They increase the space for mental health conversation and so help to reduce shame about these experiences. As a result of disclosures made by people in the public eye, it should be possible for us to say: 'If these successful, good-looking stars of sport or showbiz can feel what I feel, then maybe I shouldn't blame myself. Perhaps I shouldn't feel so ashamed.' Anything that reduces self-stigma and shame has to be good, hasn't it?

Unfortunately, while celebrity disclosure is welcome to many, there is little evidence it actually shifts common attitudes in any general sense. Indeed, our data suggests that the opposite may be true. Most people today say they are more open about mental health issues such as depression, but equally, when asked if this awareness has made them more likely to trust someone with a mental health diagnosis, they answer no. It is not clear whether this lack of trust is influenced by the specific kind of diagnosis or whether other critical factors are at play. It may be that those with a previous experience of someone with a mental health difficulty are less likely to adopt stigmatic attitudes. Awareness, it seems, is only part of the solution. Our relationship with people with mental health difficulties is also a factor.

So why don't we all just 'come out' about all our mental health challenges and acknowledge them as universal experiences within our human family? Why can't we simply stand up and declare: 'I too could have a mental health problem'? Unfortunately, disclosure by itself does not make people feel better. Indeed, disclosure may increase feelings of fear and vulnerability. At present our mental health problems may be kept in secret, but the fact that they remain secret is secondary to the real problem. Revealing our secrets does not make our problems go away. Real evidence-based therapy is required.

Other stigmatized groups have made great progress by encouraging self-disclosure, by promoting 'coming out', but I am not recommending that people come out about their mental health difficulties. My recommendation is about recovery. Recommending more self-disclosure would just expose more people to the stigmatic hostility they already fear. It is not right to ask people to tackle stigma at their peril. Martyrdom is not a legitimate anti-stigma strategy or a recovery plan, and so we cannot recommend this. It is fair to let those who can disclose do so, but for most people the perils of this approach outweigh the benefits.

Still, we can imagine it. What would happen if all the users of mental health services took the lead shown us by the celebrities and began to self-declare? The internet and social media are full of this kind of personal confession, but would stigma be reduced by more of this kind of self-declaration spilling out into the streets? Perhaps this might help us to acknowledge the universality of the mental health challenge and so we all might be less likely to see it as a problem for others, not for ourselves. After all, we understand the facts, that right at this moment every one of us has at least one family member or close relative in mental distress; every one of us knows someone with a mental health problem. Mental health problems are not just for other people, or other families, or other races, or other genders – or even other socio-economic groups: mental health difficulties intersect with everyone, everywhere.

Any truthful acknowledgement of mental health difficulty is

to be welcomed but acknowledging this is not the same as coming out. Mental health problems do not define who we are. They tell us about our human experience: things that have happened to us, and how we think, feel and behave as a result. Mental health issues are mostly transient and fluctuant. Even the more enduring common mental health problems such as schizophrenia or bipolar mood disorder should not be seen as characteristic of a human being. More education and better therapy are preferable options in the battle to defeat stigma than a campaign of self-disclosure.

Our stigmatic attitudes may arise from other sources of prejudices, however. Perhaps our misunderstanding of the difference between nature and nurture.

Nature vs Nurture: A False Dichotomy

In mental health, as in most other areas of life, black-and-white thinking seldom works. The old debate of 'nature versus nurture' is out of date. In the past, nature was wrongly seen as pre-determined, unchanging. The earliest understanding of our DNA viewed our character as fully formed at birth and as fixed as the bar codes on the groceries in our shopping trolleys. In reality, our genetic material is not so permanent. Its instructions change throughout our lifetime and they are as much subject to the environment as the other malleable aspects of our being.

The opposing perspective is also outmoded. This view regarded the force of upbringing (nurture) as all-powerful, determining and likewise unchanging, but we now know that this too is simplistic. For example, the negative effects of adverse childhood experiences are far less certain than they might appear. The data shows that most people who have experienced these events go on to find personal recovery. Our human capacity to re-shape our futures is vast. Men and women create new positive experiences for themselves and those they love, and they do this every day. This capacity for recovery is a testament to human resilience (see What Is Resilience? later in this chapter), and of our determination to heal and be healed.

21

One strength of modern mental healthcare is that these two diverse poles of thinking – nature versus nurture – are no longer separated. The best research, like the best therapy, intertwines the biological and the psychological to reveal routes to mental wellness that are holistic and inclusive. The data confirm that more than any other factor it is the social determinants of life that influence our physical and mental wellbeing.[6] These social factors also enable us to rethink the challenge of wellbeing. This 'rethinking' is part of what is known as positive psychology.

Positive Psychology

So, after all we have said, what does it really mean to be well? Perhaps no definition of our health can be entirely satisfactory. I hope by now we can agree on some things: that being healthy means more than having an absence of illness, and that there must be more to healthy living than the unattainable restoration of our youth. There may even be more to it than freedom from any particular experience, however painful. But when seen in these terms our health remains a somewhat negative construct. By contrast, positive psychologists see health as the unfettered freedom to participate in living to the full once again. From this perspective, a person's recovery from mental health problems is nothing short of their total re-engagement with life. According to this positive view, when we recover from distress, when we find wellness again, we also rediscover the fullness of life. With renewed mental wellness we rediscover our way to eat better, sleep better, play better, work better, and to love more.

Even though this positive view of wellness is attractive, there is a real danger in this kind of positive psychology. This danger is greatest when positive psychology becomes the template for the life well lived. It can be very problematic for those who are trying to recover their wellness. In difficult times the last thing we need to be presented with is a list of activities and behaviours

[6] See the Whitehall studies of Sir Michael Marmot.

that are deemed 'healthy', contrasted with a list of them deemed 'unhealthy'. It is never helpful to divide our lives into lists of good and bad. Life is about so much more than a checklist. Even a positive checklist can be a burden. The positivist attitude to wellness may just pile on more pressure to conform to yet another form of ideal.

How Can We Get Well? Talking About It Helps

Even if we could agree on what wellness looks like – if, in a sense, we could know our destination – getting there would still be a problem. It would still be a challenge for some of us. Recovery of the life well lived always involves an individual on a personal journey. The therapeutic journey always begins with a 'special' type of conversation. Defining wellness might help us to identify our goals by putting forward some great questions, but a therapeutic conversation is necessary. This is one which helps us to identify some better answers. These are the answers that relate to our challenges and to our lives. In this way, therapy tends to be less about *knowing* the way to wellness; it becomes more about *finding* our way to wellness. At this point the recovery question changes. We begin to ask, how do I get well, and how do I stay well?

Talking Therapy

All knowledge of recovery starts with such questioning. Cognitive behavioural talking therapies (to which we will bear witness in Part II) are full of these questions. Once we find the right questions, we may begin to ponder meaningful, effective answers. So, how can we agree on which questions are most helpful?

Not all questions are the same. Some may be more helpful than others. The word 'why', for example, may be less informative than it first seems. In therapy asking 'why' can lead to the past and to a series of very static answers down more intellectual and emotional cul-de-sacs. The liberating questions – the ones that open the windows to allow some air in – tend to be more current and dynamic: these are questions that begin with how, when, who, what and where. Once we ask these questions, space opens up and change is possible.

This type of questioning and reflection is not easy, of course. Especially since there are never any easy answers. Throughout this book, you will see people asking some very hard questions of themselves and about their pursuit of wellness. Every day men and women tackle these practical problems and ask themselves: How can I do all of this wellness stuff? How do I build up all of this resilience? How do I do this 'recover thing', and when and where and for how long can I do it? It is all very good trying to identify the characteristics of wellness in the abstract, but in reality these personally demanding questions remain. And how can any of us do all of this wellness stuff over and over again? One answer includes a recognition of the importance of resilience to healthy living. So what is resilience, and how can we have more of it?

What Is Resilience?

Resilience is the capacity to bounce back after distress and crucially to do this again and again. It is a vital quality and it is essential in a life lived well. Some people compare resilience to physical fitness. There is no health without mental health, as we always say, and the defining characteristic of resilience is the ability to bounce back after stress. This elasticity might be compared to an athlete's ability to recover after some extreme physical exertion.

In reality, how might resilience work for us? Many of us can recall a time when we were knocked sideways by a trauma, when sudden challenges threatened our wellbeing. We look back at events in retrospect and think that we came through them, that we were stronger in the end. But what if we didn't come through it?

Let us suppose we were to experience a time when we were truly devastated by a loss or disappointment or failure. What would we do then? Imagine it. We might have been in real mental jeopardy. Suppose the challenges to our health were even greater because in addition to our distress we were overcome by burdens of stigma, guilt and shame. And while all of this was happening to us, suppose we became dependent on a less authentic source of solace, such as alcohol or drugs. Suppose we developed some other addiction. How could we achieve wellness then? Suppose the problems were made worse still. Suppose there was no one to help us, nowhere for us to turn for help and support. How then would we maintain any of the eight dimensions of wellness? How would we maintain *any* wellness, let alone practise the 'Five Ways to Wellbeing' if in our distress we had no one to connect to, no one to be active with, no one to take notice, no one to learn from, and no one with us to give and take? What would we do then?

Over the years, many patients have told me about their individual struggles to withstand their distress and to make sense of a recovery. Sometimes they ask themselves how their crisis occurred and what led them to this vulnerable and unhappy place. Often they ask themselves why any of this pain has happened to them. Despite the fact that there may be no apparent explanation, they struggle to understand why their mental health has broken down. Blame is typical. This is one of the first things people do at a time of great stress. We blame ourselves and we blame others. In mental health distress, the burden of guilt and self-reproach is the most dangerous of all.

I always ask people if they feel their trauma was their fault, and the reply is always indicative. The self-reproachful response is typical of the depressed: 'Of course it's my fault,' they say. 'Who else is there to blame? Everything is my fault.' This posture contrasts sharply with the painful, angry reaction of the subjectively wronged. Those who blame others tend to say: 'All I want is an apology. All I want is some justice.' Both positions are frustrating. Neither is helpful. That's the thing about blame. It's useless. Of course sometimes we have to fight back. 'Don't get mad, get even', as the slogan on the bumper stickers put it. At other times, it may be more prudent to run and hide. But clinically, in times of depression, the responses to fight or take flight are just opposite ends of the same reactionary reflex. Neither response is guaranteed to build recovery. As we shall see later, neither response is actually resilient and both extremes lack compassion.

In order to regain our mental health, in order to be resilient, a broader and more liberating set of options is necessary. In the end, it is useless to blame ourselves and it may be equally useless to blame others for the stress in our life. Generating alternatives to blame is part of recovery.

Therapy, such as we shall see in this book, helps us to generate more functional responses to mental distress. These new responses are ones that go beyond the extremes of fight or flight, of shame or blame. From these renewed personal positions, recovery and resilient wellness can grow.

Emotional Resilience

Although every loss is unique our reactions to stress are always human and they are most often unconscious. That is why it is so unfair that we blame those who lose their mental health. If ever we chastise the mentally ill for their 'lack of resilience', our dismissal is counterproductive. It only increases the self-reproach of people already in distress. It affirms it in their eyes. And yet urging resilience is not the same as criticism. It is not possible for any of us to have sufficient armour to withstand every stress. Life is unpredictable and none of us knows what is around the corner.

Why not think of resilience in a different way, not as some magical form of elasticity but as a source of emotional strength to which we can return whenever we are under great stress. A resilient person is fully loaded with this deep emotional fuel. To live life well under stress we will need many sources of this resilient energy. It is from such stores that we draw our wellness. Mental illness is what happens when our emotional tank runs dry.

Psychological emptiness such as this has many causes, but adverse early childhood experience is generally regarded as one of the most significant. For the greater part of the last century, psychotherapists focused on the impact of early childhood experience and regarded this as largely determining of our adult character. The potential influence of childhood mental trauma is profound. We now know that at least three-quarters of adult mental health disorders begin before adult life is established.

We also know that many other factors contribute to wellness and so not everything is determined by our childhood years. As this more hopeful understanding of childhood experience emerged, so too a more hopeful concept of wellness grew. This is the concept of mental resilience and it owes much to the work of the English psychiatrist Sir Michael Rutter. In an interview in 2014 with the BBC for the radio programme *The Life Scientific* he talks about his childhood experience as an evacuee during the Second World War.[7] Without question, the experience left a lasting impression upon him.

Like many children at that time, the young Rutter was evacuated to safety in anticipation of the conflict. He travelled to the United States, separated from his parents, and sailed across the Atlantic Ocean at a time of real danger. Looking back on this experience caused the older Michael Rutter to question aspects of the prevailing psychological view regarding childhood trauma and maternal separation.[8]

When he recalled his own distress, as well as the distress of the other children on that wartime marine transporter, he made another observation. He noticed that not all the children were equally distressed. While every child experienced separation from their parents at a time of real wartime jeopardy, the evacuated children's distress was not homogeneous or uniform. Some children found it more difficult than others. What was the explanation for this variability? Might some children be more resilient than others, and if so why? What makes one child more resilient

---

[7] *The Life Scientific* podcasts, Sir Michael Rutter, BBC Radio 4.

[8] M. Rutter, 'Resilience in the Face of Adversity: Protective Factors and Resistance to Psychiatric Disorders', *British Journal of Psychiatry*, Vol. 147, 1995, pp. 589–611.

when stressed and another less so? Years later Rutter and his colleagues set about the study of these differences in resilient adaptability and since then many groups have sought an answer to this question. This combined study led to the modern concept we now call resilience.[9]

Today we see resilience as a process and not a single character trait, and so one model speaks of the domains of resilience.[10] We see these domains as vital sources of emotional and psychological adaptability. These are the wellsprings of emotional fuel we spoke about earlier, and they are the personal and social resources that matter when it comes to responding to stress. Rather than needing a suit of armour or the warrior strength of a Trojan, what we need when we are stressed is resilience. The more fortunate have these resources in greater abundance and they can return to these wellsprings again and again. Their resilience dimensions are like gilt-edged stocks invested in a personal bank of wellness. These are mental health riches indeed!

So, what are these six domains of resilience? They are:

- A Secure Base
- An Education
- Friendships
- Talents and Interests
- Positive Values
- Social Competence

Let's consider each of these resilience domains in turn. Are they credible? Do they make common sense? Is it plausible that these gifts would make us stronger and more likely to live life well? There can be little doubt about it. These resilient domains are like foundation stones. Each is fundamental to the project of

---

[9] Valuable information on resilience can be found at the Barnardo's UK website, www.barnardos.org.uk/bouncing_back.

[10] B. Daniel and S. Wassell, *Adolescence: Assessing and Promoting Resilience in Vulnerable Children*, Vol. 3, Jessica Kingsley, 2002.

rebuilding a life and living well. These attributes make us more prepared for the experience we call life.

And so, if we are lucky, we will have a secure base and an education as we start out and throughout life: we may have had good people to nurture us, to advise us, and to teach us a wise thing or two. We may be able to make friends – and enjoy the fact that we are social creatures after all. We may even have certain gifts of skills and talents, and we may be able to sustain positive values – seeing the value in our own lives and in the lives of others. Ultimately with these resources our mental health can grow, and we can make our way in the social world supported and sustained by our mental wellbeing. These resilient factors help us to recover our mental health – and because of these our recovered wellness becomes something to celebrate once again.

Resilient resources are not illusions or fantasies, but in reality not everyone has them all to the same level. Wellness is something we all have some investment in, but there are times when each of us could do with a bit more. The whole thrust of our education, our economy and our culture would change for the better if society fully embraced this agenda of resilient wellness. Our shared journey towards a life well lived is bound together by these common factors. These ordinary human and practical values are undeniable. Surely, it seems, we could be well?

So what must we do if, for some reason, our resilience is exhausted? What do we do then, when an overwhelming stress comes to us? Do we inevitably become 'unwell'? This brings me to another very familiar question: What exactly is a mental health disorder anyway?

2

What Does It Mean to Have a Mental Health Diagnosis?

OUR DISCUSSION OF WELLNESS is all very fine, as far as it goes, but it still leaves us with some very big unanswered questions about illness and about how to live well after it. When all is said and done, what is a mental illness? What, if anything, is achieved by diagnosing and labelling it as one? To put this question more sharply, we might ask this: What is the use of making a diagnosis in mental health?

Most people agree about the value of diagnosis in other areas of medicine, such as infectious diseases or cancers. Here a diagnosis can help to clarify the experience by providing a common language for it, so that we can all understand and examine it further. A useful diagnosis may even describe the cause of a disease, as well as charting the course of its treatment. Making such a medical diagnosis enables us to communicate a predictable outcome of an illness and it can guide us towards the best management. Unfortunately, this is where the problem with mental health diagnosis arises. You see, diagnoses in mental health don't really do much of this good stuff!

From the beginning of time, physicians have addressed the problem of illness from this same starting point. So doctors make diagnoses, and it is clear why we do. A good diagnosis is very helpful for the physician – and hopefully good for the patient as well. The therapeutic approach to illness based upon diagnosis is known as 'the medical model'. Unfortunately, mental health diagnoses lack this predictive or therapeutic medical value. And when they are used to predict management in this way a great deal of harm may be done.

Take, for example, the great nineteenth-century neuro-psychiatrist Emil Kraepelin. He was one of the most famous diagnosticians in the world and his most notable diagnosis was one he called 'dementia praecox'. He used this term to describe a condition seen in young men or women who experienced a profound mental breakdown or psychosis. This psychosis was typically associated with abnormal perceptions known as hallucinations (or hearing voices when no one is there). The same condition was later renamed schizophrenia, but the term 'dementia praecox' is important for this reason. Kraepelin's dementia concept implied a brain disorder with a prediction of inevitable decline. Fortunately, nothing could have been further from the truth. The outcome of psychoses such as schizophrenia is more varied than Kraepelin ever imagined. Many people given this diagnosis today make a very positive recovery.

Unfortunately, the 'dementia praecox' concept became stuck in our consciousness despite the evidence to the contrary. Much of our persistent pessimism about mental health is explained by this negativity. That is why making a diagnosis is such a significant problem in mental health. Our labels do not have much predictive value. They tell us nothing about causes and very little about cures. Even when they are made reliably they simply help us to talk to each other about some experiences that we would otherwise be silent about.

So why do we still make diagnoses? Partly because a diagnosis provides professionals with a clear language to communicate important information – about patterns of behaviour and about our response to them. We need to study these phenomena and we can only do this if they are reliably described. The predictive value of classification may be questionable, but there is nothing served by abandoning descriptive diagnosis altogether. There is no point in throwing the proverbial baby out with the bathwater!

ICD or DSM?

To understand just how the diagnostic process works in the real world, let me first explain that there are two standard diagnostic systems used in the western world. In Europe, we use the International Classification of Disease (ICD), published by the World Health Organization (WHO). In the USA, mental health services use the Diagnostic and Statistical Manual (DSM), published by the American Psychiatric Association (APA). Such is the interest in and controversy surrounding these systems that a new edition of the DSM manual is likely to make the cover of *Time* magazine!

The point is that these systems of diagnosis are actually perfectly formed. They do exactly what they say on the tin. In other words, they do what they were intended to do. They reliably produce diagnoses (or descriptions) of common major mental health problems, such as schizophrenia and depression, and many others besides. Nowadays, because these descriptions are agreed, a condition such as schizophrenia diagnosed in London is exactly the same condition as that diagnosed in New York or Rome or Moscow. So the ICD and DSM are undoubtedly reliable systems, and this reliability allows for a more consistent dialogue about the incidence and prevalence of mental health problems across the whole globe.

The ICD and DSM both work in a list-wise fashion by ranking numbers of symptoms to make a total picture that informs the diagnosis. To see how it operates, it is probably best to look at the criteria used for a common diagnosis such as depression.

The tenth edition of the ICD Instruction Manual uses an agreed list of ten depressive symptoms in order to make a diagnosis of depression. Three symptoms are key. They are persistent sadness or lowered mood, loss of interests or pleasure, and fatigue or loss of energy. At least one of these must be present most days and most of the time for at least two weeks. If one of them is present, the diagnostician must enquire about seven other features. These symptoms are disturbed sleep, poor concentration or indecisiveness, low self-confidence, poor or increased appetite, suicidal thoughts or acts, agitation or slowing of movements, and guilt or self-blame. Together these ten symptoms define the degree of depression. Those with fewer than four symptoms are deemed not to be depressed. Those with four symptoms and only four should be diagnosed with mild depression. Those with five or six symptoms have moderate depression. Those with seven or more symptoms have severe depression, with or without psychotic symptoms (whether or not they have lost touch with reality). Severe depression is diagnosed when the symptoms are present for four weeks or more and all the symptoms are experienced daily.

As you can see, the diagnosis is based on the presence or absence of numbers of symptoms. But what if the person has more than one mental health problem at the same time? A diagnosis based on a list of symptoms might tell us something about the length of a particular problem, but it tells us nothing about its breadth. So how do these systems operate when a person has a more complex problem?

Actually, the chances of having another problem are very high and so it's important that every diagnosis is fully recognized, especially complex or multiple ones. Many people with depression have an overlapping set of problems with coexistent difficulties, such as anxiety disorder, obsessive compulsive disorder, phobic disorder or post-traumatic stress disorder. By adding list-wise the criteria for any number of these problems, ICD or DSM systems build up a more useful two-dimensional picture of a person's problem. This way the diagnosis ends up looking like an overlapping set of coordinates. It becomes more like a map than a single label.

Descriptions such as these are useful. In some ways they are invaluable. This is especially so once we agree on their purpose – simply to describe experience and to do this reliably. In this regard, we might take the advice of the great philosopher Ludwig Wittgenstein, who advised that we should 'only describe, don't explain'. When ICD or DSM is used in this descriptive way, mental health diagnoses are worthwhile because they allow us to communicate in an objective way.

Gardening

To illustrate the value of this point let's think about the issue of diagnosis in another way. Take gardening, for example. Suppose there was an ICD or DSM of flowers, shrubs and trees. Using this imaginary ICD or DSM, we could reliably list species and highlight potential diseases within each category. This imaginary ICD or DSM gardening edition would be a fantastic resource for someone interested in categorizing the diseases of all known plants. Nevertheless, this knowledge alone would not tell us how to grow a thriving plant. It is simply an identifier of a class. It tells us little about the individual daffodil or oak. The categorical gardener still needs to find out where to plant it and how to make it grow. An accurate description of plants in the garden won't answer these gardening questions, though it might be a good place to start.

The therapeutic gardener needs to know much more. The meaningful questions about growth and prosperity remain. What is the best way to help each flower, shrub or tree to reach its full potential? The categorical description of the garden won't in itself tell us anything about this.

Is Treatment Determined by Diagnosis?

So, what does all this descriptive diagnostic stuff do for those of us in real distress? What does it tell us about the decision to recommend a therapy? What factors determine the best mental health treatment? How does the recommended treatment relate to diagnosis? To answer these questions, it's worth considering what the ideal therapy might look like. Given all we have said, you might expect me to say that the best treatment is simply one that is based upon a particular description of the problems (a diagnosis). Surely this diagnostic description must form the basis for an ideal plan of care? Unfortunately in mental health nothing is that simple.

Medication vs Therapy: Which Is Best?

There are times when medication is appropriate. It is fair to say that as a doctor I may prescribe medication either on its own or in conjunction with other aspects of treatment, including therapy. Although this book will not dwell on these prescriptions at length, it is only fair to say that medication is not a lesser form of treatment or necessarily a less effective one. For many people, medication may be a beneficial and even essential part of treatment. Neither are people who take medication in any way less deserving of respect or kindness. The right question to ask is this: What treatment is in the best interest of each man or woman in mental distress? If the best care includes medication, then so be it. If it includes the combination of medication *and* therapy, and if the person is fully informed as to the risks and benefits of every aspect of treatment, then it is only right to recommend such a combination. It's about the person in distress.

Three things should underpin the ideal choice of therapy. These are:

1. Full clinical assessment of the patient
2. Good evidence of the proposed treatment's effectiveness
3. Genuinely informed consent of the patient

When it comes to the choice of psychotherapy, there is no 'one size fits all' treatment, and there is no universal 'best' route to recovery. This clinical complexity is part of the challenge of recovery, and it arises from the sheer heterogeneity of human beings and the infinite variety of their mental health problems.

We know that diagnostic systems produce reliable, consistent labels. That's what they are designed to do. By contrast, therapy responds to an almost limitless variety of individual human difficulties. When offered in this personal way, therapy becomes more individually engaging and therefore more effective than any diagnostic label could ever have predicted.

To illustrate this individual aspect of therapy, let's imagine choosing a therapy for one hundred people with a diagnosis of clinical depression. Even if each of these people had the same diagnosis, each would have a different story, arising in a different social context and from a different set of life experiences. One hundred diagnoses may be the same, but the context and the triggers for each personal crisis will still be unique. Similarly, although human beings may experience the same degrees of distress, we all find different ways to recover. That is why there are as many different recovery stories as there are stars in the sky. And since there are many different routes to recovery there are also many different estimates of the value of recovery. While some people feel they have already made sufficient 'progress' and so consider themselves recovered, others may remain genuinely disappointed and feel that their recovery falls way short of what they were entitled to expect.

So you see, here you have a crucial difference in mental health. Diagnoses may strive for descriptive objectivity and reliability, but the engagement with therapy is always subjective and each relationship is unique. What is more, while mental health diagnoses are made in an objective, clinical context, the real men and women in distress still experience mental health problems in their own personal context. In this natural environment many complex social forces are at play. Environmental, biological, psychological, spiritual and even political factors may be involved.

This subjectivity makes mental health problems very human and very real. That is why mental health problems are better understood as 'social constructs' experienced and recognized by us in the real world. They are defined most valuably in two arenas, within the person and within society. In this context mental health problems become more than two-dimensional clinical labels derived from lists of symptoms: they are three-dimensional subjective problems experienced in ordinary life.

All of this has been recognized by those concerned with the development of modern therapy. To a great extent, each therapy described in this book deals less with clinical diagnosis than with real, three-dimensional, unique human challenges. These therapies are about helping people recover real human, social and interpersonal functions. To put it another way, if mental health therapy was a movie, clinical diagnostics might be in 2D, but therapy would have to be in 3D.

So, Which Therapy?

Excellent mental healthcare depends on human resources and so it requires skilled therapeutic labour. Unfortunately, the choice of therapies offered to most patients still falls far short of the ideal. Choice of therapy, where it exists, is very limited. Even though mental healthcare should be a societal priority, it is not resourced as such. Even though our human rights should determine it, they do not. Every person should have a right to fully participate in their recovery, but this right requires choice. Sadly, for most people choice simply does not exist. Mental healthcare providers do their best for the majority of people, and most of the time most do it with very limited resources. As a result, none of the factors we have discussed is actually what determines the offering of therapy. Neither diagnosis nor therapeutic evidence nor human rights in the end has much bearing on the choice of effective therapy.

What Determines the Choice of Therapy?

Whether someone is offered a therapy or not comes down to three things. These are what we sometimes call the three 'A's. They are access, availability and affordability. These are the real factors that predict whether your care plan or mine will include excellent, effective modern therapy within a human-rights framework.

Let's take a closer look. None of these factors is determined in any way by the diagnosis or the content of a person's problem. And it would be wrong to suggest that the problem of therapy is just about resources – there are never enough resources. But there is more to it than that. Access to therapy is about the definition of the mental health problems as well.

To illustrate this, let us suppose we were in an ideal world.

Suppose real and effective therapies were available in an open, transparent and non-judgemental environment. Let's go even further and imagine that there were sufficient numbers of trained therapists available with all the skills to maximize the benefits of each treatment. And let's suppose that in this ideal world patients were able and willing to fully engage with therapy from the start. For me, this would be therapeutic heaven. But what then? How would therapy work in such an ideal world?

In these ideal circumstances the choice of therapy would be influenced not by a diagnosis but by the individual emotional and behavioural needs of each man or woman seeking help. Others might say that a diagnosis is a description of those needs, but in truth the emotional, mental and behavioural needs of human beings extend far beyond specific mental health labels. These trans-diagnostic issues include fear and anger, grief and shame, and so they transcend our current concept of mental health diagnosis. Sometimes these transcendent issues include behaviours such as avoidance and addiction. Sometimes they include other errors of thinking, as well as behaviours, and sometimes even include risks of self-harm and suicidality.

These problems are real mental health difficulties recognized by men and women seeking help. They occur in real life and they straddle all the diagnoses. They may be described as trans-diagnostic issues because they are universal and human; they are not confined to or defined by any particular diagnosis. Even in an ideal world these issues would be central to a genuine therapeutic care plan. In an ideal world these issues would be the first things addressed. And so only when these issues are addressed can the effectiveness of therapy become truly apparent.

In short, categorical diagnoses – descriptive labels in accordance with manuals such as the ICD and DSM – form only part of the clinical picture, a two-dimensional part at best. When we listen to patients and respond to their transcendent emotions, then mental healthcare becomes more humane and less reliant on categorical labels. It is then that we realize that people are three-dimensional and not flat.

This goes some way to explain why this book will not focus on treatments for particular diagnoses such as phobias, eating disorders, depression, alcohol-dependence syndrome, post-traumatic stress disorder or borderline personality. Even though my patients have all of these problems, and many others besides, none of these diagnostic labels determines or limits the benefits of the particular therapies I wish to describe. Put simply, useful therapy responds to human beings and not to diagnoses. Therapy is about the issues that make all our lives more difficult – by responding to these problems, modern therapy hopes to make this recovery journey more positive and more sustained.

I suspect (although I cannot prove this) that the effectiveness of the therapies referenced in this book arises for this reason. All legitimate forms of modern therapy aim to help people recover, but the modern therapy described here does this by helping people to overcome fears and anger, grief and shame, along with many other human manifestations of mental distress and difficulty.

In my experience, men and women engage best when mental healthcare is relevant and meaningful to them, when it is appropriate to their experiences and their needs. Therapeutic engagement becomes possible because its finally in therapy that we address this whole human agenda. A more humane focus means the work of recovery may also be engaging.

So, what does a modern recovery journey look like – and what exactly are these modern therapies? We shall take a look at these later when we meet the patients whose recoveries we will describe, but before we do that we need to understand a little about them. It is necessary to look back at the therapies from which these modern forms grew, specifically Behaviour Therapy (BT) and Cognitive Behavioural Therapy (CBT).

3

Recovery and the Good Life: The Origins of Modern Therapy

W E BELIEVE THAT WE can be well. To be precise, we believe that we can learn to live and love and work again. This is our mantra, so it is more than an aspiration. It is a faith in our potential for recovery. Of course you may dismiss this declaration as nothing more than a dream or the re-statement of a wish, but is this optimism just self-deception? Is there evidence to support our therapeutic credo? Is it really possible to learn to live well again?

The pursuit of a better life persists, and it does so in the real world despite all its problems. Recovery is contingent on very many factors – on nature and circumstance and many powerful dynamics in the environment. Many of these forces are beyond our control. It would be facile to dismiss the unforeseen influence of chance. Life is full of randomness, and dumb luck may be a factor for good or ill. Despite our best intentions, and even in the most advantageous circumstances, a man or woman may be cut down too early by a bullet coming right out of the blue. 'The best-laid plans of mice and men', as they say.

Still, our belief in the achievement of wellness is sustained by more than hope. It is supported by compelling evidence confirming the existence of many restorative human abilities. Paramount among these is our ability to learn. Human beings can learn and we do so every day. This learning is the basis of our capacity to adapt and to live life well again. Modern psychotherapy has captured this human learning and harnessed it in new and more effective ways. Modern therapy (including the therapies I have chosen to highlight in this book) places supreme emphasis on the value of learning.

Unfortunately, therapy is still widely misunderstood. Many people still view the experience of going to a therapist as somewhere between the confessional and the court room. Actually real therapy has little in common with these travesties and its agenda is neither confessional nor judgemental. Modern therapy is about human discovery. At its core it is about the search for a way to live well again. Obviously many factors contribute to the efficacy of this therapy. Compassionate listening and empathy must be there, but my hope is that through these stories you will see that modern psychotherapy offers much more than relaxation and support. Modern therapy provides an opportunity for learning that is meaningful and full of potential.

I am not suggesting that any of the new therapies in this book arose *de novo* or without reference to significant past contributions, but it is not my purpose to summarize the history of psychotherapy or to attempt to do justice to giants such as Freud and Jung or their successors. Neither will I discuss at length any of psychotherapy's many debts to Buddhism or Judaism, Christianity or Stoicism – or any other seminal cultural set. It is beyond my scope to go into the background of these influences, save only to acknowledge that these influences do exist.

It is necessary to go into more detail about two particular therapies. These are Behaviour Therapy and its successor Cognitive Behavioural Therapy. I will refer frequently to their use throughout this book and in order to understand the new therapeutic paths highlighted here it is essential that we discuss these two in detail for a moment.

So, What Is Behaviour Therapy?

Behaviour Therapy (BT) is a long-established form of psychotherapy based on a learning phenomenon known as 'conditioning'. Many of the visceral and cerebral experiences associated with fear are actually responsive to conditioning. We can learn to overcome symptoms such as anxiety, palpitations and sweating, even the fear of death, all so typical of panic disorder, because these problems are all amenable to conditioning. These fear sensations can be reconditioned through an element of BT called 'exposure' – specifically exposure to the feared stimulus. This BT is especially helpful when it is associated with the prevention of avoidance.

Over time distressing and disabling bodily responses diminish in BT and, what is more, the beneficial effects are cumulative. The fearful symptoms reduce even more in response to further exposure to the same stimulus. To put it simply, behavioural psychotherapy capitalizes on the body's natural tendency to adapt to things. BT reconditions us to overcome things that previously disturbed or disabled us.

The origins of Behaviour Therapy lie in the work of the great Russian neuropsychiatrist Ivan Pavlov in the late nineteenth century. Since then BT has developed, supported by vast psychological research. Its efficacy cannot be denied. BT focuses primarily on conditioning our feelings and sensations, but it has very little to say directly about our thoughts or our beliefs. It acts in two ways, by adapting our visceral reactions and by challenging our avoidant responses. In time, these visceral reactions are reduced or toned down, and so our responses find new, less distressing and less disabling levels. As our avoidance declines experience shows that we become more engaged with life and start to live well again.

BT is an effective treatment for a wide range of mental health difficulties, such as agoraphobia, specific phobia and panic disorder. Although its value has been recognized for decades, its advocates grew silent in the wake of progress made by newer therapies such as Cognitive Behavioural Therapy (CBT). Even more recent advances have reaffirmed the fundamental value of BT. In effect, the therapeutic benefit of two of its key elements has been rediscovered. These are the elements known as 'exposure' and 'response prevention'.

The modern therapies described later in this book include treatments such as Compassion Focused Therapy (CFT) and Dialectical Behaviour Therapy (DBT). These new forms of therapy brought the practical restorative benefit of BT back into focus. It remains an effective method since it teaches us new ways to respond to our experiences and new ways of doing something about them. BT has become an invaluable part of the modern wellness tool box.

Still, as we have said, Behaviour Therapy has less to say about what we think and more to do with how we behave. There is nothing abstract or obscure about its path to wellness. Like most modern therapies it focuses on the 'here and now'. It is really only concerned with the present. Its methods are about learning to experience stress differently and behave differently in response. The enduring appeal of BT comes from its success in teaching these new ways to experience and behave. All of this means that BT can be a dramatically effective and measurable part of the pathway to wellness.

Sarah's Story

To illustrate Behaviour Therapy, let me tell you about one of my very first patients, a woman I saw when I was a young psychiatrist-in-training at the Maudsley Hospital in London.

Her name was Sarah and she had an overwhelming anxiety caused by her fear of contamination. Sarah was terrified of animal faeces, particularly dog faeces. As a result, she experienced crippling levels of anxious tension in many areas of her life. Caring for her despite her fearful experience taught me so much about what life is like for those gripped by visceral fear and by almost total avoidance of life.

One of the most troubling features of these anxiety problems tends to be the long delay people experience before getting effective help. On average people wait more than ten whole years before they engage with an effective therapy for an anxiety disorder. This is remarkable since we now know that panic anxieties and phobias are readily responsive to BT. Its principal interventions, Exposure and Response Prevention (ERP), are powerful tools and there is no reason to delay applying them.

Obviously her fear was no trivial matter for Sarah. She had been anxious and avoidant for many years. Fear dominated her daily life. Yet her successful treatment using BT did not involve any exhaustive discussion on the sources of her fear of dog faeces. Neither did she go through any lengthy psychological speculation as to the causes of her preoccupation with it. Sarah's experience was taken for what it was in the 'here and now'. It was taken at face value, non-judgementally. Sarah's problem was acknowledged. She was a woman trapped by fear. Our care plan was to recondition her fear response and so set her free.

In my naivety, I expected that I might have to expose Sarah to large amounts of dog faeces in our clinic. Privately, I was wary at the prospect of being the one to go and collect the stuff in large amounts. Such tasks usually fall to the most junior on the multi-disciplinary team! To my great relief, the team decided that exposure for Sarah could be more easily achieved by simply taking her for a walk in the park located near the hospital on Denmark Hill in South London. My instructions were to take Sarah to Ruskin Park and to stay with her there while she was exposed to her fears. And so began my first experience of a successful BT.

As we walked together Sarah spoke at length about her wish to make progress and to overcome the fear that was holding her back.

'It's not as if I haven't tried before to get over this stuff. I've read book after book,' she said. 'And I've taken all kinds of advice. And I do know it's a stupid thing really. My fear is so stupid. But it's all-powerful and it's everywhere. Dog poo, for goodness sake! It could be anywhere! So I can't take any chances. It may be daft to you, but it has always seemed very real and dangerous to me. I can't take any risks with this.'

Understanding Sarah's fear is helpful. Fear behaves just as Sarah described it. Fear spreads, and we call this spreading of fear phenomenon 'generalization'. Fear extends beyond physical limits and so in the end a fear that may once have been local and limited is to be found everywhere. In the same way, the response to fear also generalizes. Sarah's avoidant response is audible: she insists she 'can't take any risks'. This posture leads her to avoidance and as this behaviour extends it becomes a dominant feature. We call this 'phobic anxiety'. It is such a common disability and affects up to four in every hundred of the community.

In our modern world, the phenomenon of fear generalization is not sufficiently understood. There are some who thrive on it and they really understand how it works: these are the terrorists. When these fear-makers plant bombs and commit atrocities intending to terrorize us, they use fear. And so an attack such as at the Bataclan Theatre in Paris becomes a possibility anywhere in Paris and at any theatre in the world. The terrorists spread fear; in effect, they generalize it. This is why the impact of any terror event can extend, crossing borders and moving around the world.

Unwittingly, our modern twenty-four-hour news media contributes to this generalization of anxiety with its flash head-lines and fifteen-minute updates of every global atrocity. Once the fear generalizes, the terrorists have their wish: not only have they made victims out of their immediate targets but they have also unleashed terror on the wider community. Terrorists understand how fear generalizes; they know how it spreads. The terrorists' real aim is to spread this particular psychological toxin and with it to paralyse as many lives as possible.

And yet paralysing fear does not only arise with terrorist attacks. As we have seen in Sarah's case, it can begin with some-thing as commonplace as dog poo. At first, Sarah may have been just a little bit more sensitive about the substance than most other people, but once her fear took hold it grew and so did her phobic behaviour, her avoidance. A vicious cycle formed: this same fear of dog poo became her personal prison. Through nearly a decade of avoidance, a life that had once been full and engaged became narrow and constricted. When she came to us, she was almost completely isolated.

Sarah and I talked more about her experiences as we walked together in the park in South London. Although Sarah remained vigilant and on the alert, she walked on none the less.

By our third 'outing' (as Sarah called them), she was a little less apprehensive, but her attitude was still sceptical and she was inclined to minimize her progress.

'This can't be therapy,' she said. 'I mean, you can't really be serious? This is not what I expected you would recommend when you said you could help me to get well again. I would never have walked here unless you had suggested it and unless you had agreed to come along with me. Do you know, I wasn't always a scaredy cat?'

Sarah talked more about her fears. 'I was always a bit fussy about things, but no fussier than many people. Eventually this "fear" thing just took a grip of me and even I could see that it was getting worse. My whole body would shake. I felt very anxious and short of breath, and then I would be sure I was going to die. I suppose I didn't notice my world coming to a stop until it did, and then for no reason that I can pinpoint I just couldn't go out any more. I couldn't function outside my home. I felt trapped. I'm lucky I've a good brother. We keep in touch, him and me, and he always keeps a link with me when things get bad.'

Quite suddenly, as we were walking and talking, a large dog came running towards us off the leash. It barked and jumped about in pursuit of a ball that had been thrown towards us by its owner. As we walked on, another small dog stopped and then it defecated right in front of us on the side of the path. It must have seemed to Sarah that dogs and their mess were all around her. She became visibly frightened and upset. Later she told me that at that moment she feared she might collapse and die. She said her heart was pounding and she felt trapped because she knew she couldn't run away. Then she experienced the full-blown panic attack she had been dreading for so long.

'I felt suddenly breathless,' she said, 'as though I was going to choke. It was as if my life was coming to an abrupt end. But then something else remarkable happened. My heartbeat began to settle, my breathing eased and I realized I wasn't dying. That's the strange thing. It was an awful experience, but I survived. And even though I was fearful and upset, I didn't feel I had totally failed.'

'How did you get through it?' I asked.

'It helped me that I could see that you were not distressed. Somehow I was able to copy your behaviour and my heart started to calm down. Afterwards, I felt completely exhausted and very strange. I don't know whether this makes any sense, but somehow I knew that I had not been defeated and so I felt able to carry on.'

And Sarah did go on. Over three more walks Sarah faced her anxiety again and each time she learned more about how to overcome her dread feelings. It wasn't at all easy for her. At times she was very anxious and fearful, but overall she experienced less distress each time we walked. On our last outing, we talked about her next steps.

'I suppose I can't expect my therapist to come for a walk with me everywhere I go, can I?'

'No, Sarah. I don't think that would work.'

'Well, then, there is nothing for it. I know what I think I will have to do.'

'What's that?'

'Maybe I'll get myself my own little dog. Who would ever have thought I would say something like that?'

'I would. I always believed you could get well.'

'Maybe you did. I guess. It seems a bit ironic, I know, but it's not unreasonable. After all, they have guide dogs for the blind. I could have a pet dog for my fears. I'll call him my therapy dog.'

We both laughed as we continued to talk about Sarah's plans for the future, then we made our final walk back to the clinic before saying goodbye.

Sarah's anxiety diminished as she responded to the feared situation with a new behaviour. This new positive action was distinctly different from her former panic anxiety and avoidance. She had observed someone else who did not experience panic or fear, and who did not wish to run away. We call this BT process 'modelling'. Sarah learned to reduce her anxiety response and to stay with the feared experience and, ultimately, to overcome it. Rather than succumbing to avoidance, she became reconditioned to new and healthy experiences and responses. This hopeful rediscovery was captured elegantly in the bestselling book by Susan Jeffers, *Feel the Fear and Do It Anyway*.

Sarah also rediscovered another resilient source of wellness – her sense of humour. To this day, I don't know if she ever got her little therapy dog but through therapy she certainly learned to laugh again and that was something she had not done in a very long time.

Sarah engaged with BT using ERP and so her recovery involved a readily observable objective change. This measurable evidence of change is one of the most powerful strengths of BT. It delivers real evidence of success in problems such as panic and avoidance, and so (for those who fully engage) it is a relatively rapid and objective source of symptom relief.

The early advocates of BT found themselves in possession of vast data demonstrating tangible effectiveness. Their data probably gave them a considerable sense of superiority over other therapists and their predecessors. Disagreements about therapy of all kinds peaked at this time, when disputes about the direction of mental healthcare in general were also at their height. Unfortunately, the potential advance of therapeutic progress was delayed for years by bitter arguments between warring schools of therapeutic practice. These battles, known as 'the psych wars', did little to progress mental healthcare or widen access to therapy.

Psychiatry in Dissent

Before modern therapy could take the next step forward, another mental healthcare revolution happened. This revolution involved the total dismantlement of the asylum system across the western world. It is not my task to summarize this history here since this has been written about in many other places. It is sufficient to say this: over the next half-century the mental healthcare asylum system went into liquidation. During this time a war of words between various schools of psychiatric thought continued and as these rows progressed they became ever more personal and uncompromising.

Doubtless the revolution was necessary. There was an urgent need to end institutional care in which vast numbers of people had been incarcerated. The asylums had become swollen beyond justification. Many patients confined to these places were abandoned and some were simply forgotten. While therapeutic despair was prominent in most quarters, elsewhere ever more extreme and hazardous treatments were being prescribed. All this happened in an era before objective research and so many of these measures were introduced without sufficient evidence. Examples of such drastic medical interventions include insulin coma therapy and frontal lobotomy brain surgery. These extreme treatments were of little or no enduring benefit to their patients. Their consequences for patients' lives and wellbeing were a lasting source of discredit to the psychiatric establishment. Talking treatments were also seen as problematic. There was a growing frustration with the length of time needed for some psychological treatments. These seemed to provide an inefficient route towards humane recovery. Radical thinkers such as R. D. Laing and Thomas Szasz even questioned the existence of mental illness. Szasz went so far as to declare mental illness 'a myth', while Laing reconsidered the diagnosis of schizophrenia as a consequence of man's inhumanity to man.

As a result, throughout the second half of the twentieth century and to the present day mental healthcare remains in a state of flux. Attempts to achieve coherence have been few.[1] Instead, bitter argument persists, with extremes expressed on every side.

The Mind–Body Divide

Of course the conflicts underlying the psychiatric wars were not new. Some of these divisions have very deep roots. They arise from much older philosophical divisions, dating back to the beginnings of the Enlightenment. Principal among these is the entirely false division of the mind from the body. Sadly, belief in this

1 A. Clare, *Psychiatry in Dissent: Controversial Issues in Thought and Practice*, Routledge, 1976.

50

division persists in our public consciousness. It contributes to many persistent polarized debates about science and human understanding. On the one hand there are those who believe that knowledge of life (and by extension of the mind) comes only from scientific experiment. On the other hand there are those who argue that science can never fully explain all of human mental experience. Modern science is seen by some of its supporters as an all-powerful tool, while others see the scientific method as still lacking when it comes to the study of life. Questions as to why we live and why we love, questions that are integral to understanding human behaviour, seem for some beyond more narrowly defined boundaries of empirical scientific medicine.

Sadly, the mental healthcare debate remains polarized today. The truth is as ever somewhere in the middle. Objectively speaking, behaviourism represented some scientific progress since it showed that many aspects of human behaviour could be treated in a scientific way, but even this progress left many questions unanswered. Behavioural recovery goes only so far, and not so far as to address deeper questions about what it is to think and live life well. What was needed was a new psychology, one that extended beyond our visceral senses to include the thinking parts of the mind. This was the new psychology that gave us Cognitive Behavioural Therapy.

Cognitive Behavioural Therapy (CBT)

The new generation of cognitive therapists acknowledged their debt to Behaviour Therapy, but they also recognized its limitations. As they saw it, BT lacked the ability to achieve more than an understanding of panic and avoidance. The new cognitive behavioural therapists had a greater ambition: to develop a new therapy that went far beyond their predecessors by reaching for the parts of the mind and human life that BT could not reach.

Cognitive Behavioural Therapy (CBT) concerns itself with thoughts, beliefs, feelings and behaviours. Within CBT all of these phenomena are seen as linked, and so undoing mental distress through CBT is about more than modifying a single learned behaviour or visceral reflex. It is about learning to integrate new thoughts and new learning with new emotional responses. The question for CBT is this: Can thoughts and beliefs be modified through learning? We know that behaviours can be modified through a form of learning, but can the same be true for thoughts?

The compelling evidence came from Aaron T. Beck and his peers (the originators of CBT for depression). Human beings can learn to change their thinking and this learning brings about relief of symptoms for many people with depression and anxiety.[2] The CBT community published their results in many scientific journals and soon this data was replicated around the world.

The early data proved that CBT is an effective treatment not only for depression but also for anxiety disorders. Recently less successful attempts have been made to demonstrate its effectiveness for problems such as bipolar mood and in psychosis. CBT modifies thoughts and anxieties as well as bodily responses and behaviours. Each of these benefits increases as therapeutic progress continues. These specific recoveries generalize and as a result an extensive recovery becomes possible. To understand CBT in general, let's look at CBT for depression in a little more detail.

CBT for Depression

Beck proposed that a triad of issues dominate our psychological view. These issues involve concerns regarding our self, our future and our world. Identifying how our thoughts, beliefs, sensations and behaviours are connected can help us to understand these links and thereby learn how to address them. Identifying these thoughts provides a new target for therapy.

It's important to be clear about what we mean by 'depression'.

[2] A. T. Beck and D. J. Dozois, 'Cognitive Therapy: Current Status and Future Directions', *Annual Review of Medicine*, Vol. 62, 2011, pp. 397–409, doi: 10.1146/annurev-med-052209-100032.

When we speak of depression, we mean a persistent lowering of mood associated with subjective feelings of loss of joy, loss of energy and loss of hope. It is a very common problem. The best figures indicate that more than twenty million people in Europe are currently experiencing a clinically significant depression. One in five of our population will have an episode of depression at some stage in their lifetime.

Of course, this depression has many manifestations, and some have both subjective and objective aspects. These include loss of concentration and loss of motivation, loss of appetite and loss of weight. Consequently, it is difficult to divide depression into aspects that are entirely open to modification by learning and others that are not, but everyone agrees that depression involves three main interrelated areas, which are:

- Reduced mental activity (negative thinking)
- Altered physical activity
- Impairment of judgement

In the past it was assumed that the negative thinking seen in depression was primarily caused by the lowering of mood. In other words, it was believed that lowering of mood came first. Beck made a counter-intuitive proposal. He suggested that the reverse was actually true. What if the primary problem in depression was negative thinking? What if each of the other features – biological, psychological and social – was secondary to negative thinking? Once this model was proposed it opened up a whole new avenue for psychological research and treatment. If depressed thinking was primary, could it be learned, and did it also follow that it could be unlearned?

When Beck described these negative thoughts, he called them 'systemic errors of thinking'. He proposed these errors were the primary basis for some forms of the depressive experience. Beck described them and he named them as selective attention to the negative features of a situation, magnification of the cata-strophic implications of a situation, and what he called 'arbitrary inferences' – pessimistic conclusions drawn from a situation without any reference to the reality of any given situation.

Beck went on to propose that depressive patterns of thinking can give rise to a 'negative triad': a bleak and despairing perspective on the self, the future and the world. According to this theory, depression can lock a person into this triad with negative automatic thoughts (NATs). These errors of thinking are persistent because of even deeper beliefs that Beck and others have since called 'cognitive schema'. These schema form the basis from which NATs emerge, and from which they persist and recur.

To understand all of this, let's take a moment to think about our mood. Each of us has a belief system. These beliefs help us to organize and govern ourselves, and also to organize and govern our perceptions and behaviours. Many of our deeply held beliefs (schemas) are helpful, but others may not be so constructive. A helpful schema might be this: 'Whenever I work hard, I can usually solve most of my problems.' An unhelpful schema might be this: 'It doesn't matter what I do in life, the dice will always be loaded against me.' Beck proposed that certain critical incidents in our life can activate our dysfunctional schema. This is more likely when our negative assumptions appear to be congruent with critical negative events. This toxic convergence results in depression through a surge in our NATs, with all their associated negative emotions and feelings. According to Beck, the result is depression of our mood.

Beck's cognitive theory of depression, with all its references to negative triads, NATs and cognitive schema, would have been of little value if it remained a theory. It would have remained jargon and nothing else. What made Beck's work on depression so important was the research into therapy that emerged from it. The subsequent explosion of research into clinical practice and CBT changed the delivery of care for many people. This research did more than test his theory, it demonstrated that depressive thinking errors could be learned and unlearned. Research confirmed the effectiveness of CBT for depression.

Studies showed that when depressed patients are helped to

recognize their NATs, they discover they are able to challenge them. Just as Behaviour Therapy helped people to challenge negative behaviours, Cognitive Behavioural Therapy helped depressed patients to replace their NATs with more realistic and appropriate thoughts. More helpful thoughts and feelings could also be learned.

Many of the exposure techniques of BT are readily adaptable to CBT. Patients are encouraged to keep a diary (a 'cognitive diary') and to carry out behavioural experiments (exposure) in the real world in order to test the validity of their thoughts and perceptions. This exposure encouraged people to observe their activity, to acknowledge their successes as well as their failures, and to appreciate the joy and relief of a less negative experience of the self and the world.

Put simply, the success of CBT revealed this truth: what we think about our situation matters. Our health depends upon more than just what we do. Wellness also depends on how we think, especially on how we think about our future, ourselves and the world around us. When the CBT researchers studied the mindset of patients with depression, their work demonstrated that errors of thinking could be challenged and they could be unlearned. Toxic beliefs could be replaced with new, more constructive, healthy ways of thinking. Wellness could be restored once healthy thoughts were adopted mentally and incorporated into our way of thinking.

Unfortunately, as things turned out, CBT didn't work for every patient or for every complex problem – just as BT did not work for every patient or every problem behaviour. This stands to reason. There is no 'one size fits all' solution to mental health problems. And there were other problems. The duration of therapy was also an issue. Some saw therapy as too short, others too long. Many people dropped out or abandoned therapy and these issues were more of a problem when BT or CBT techniques were applied rigidly or narrowly.

In time the demand grew for a more egalitarian, more holistic treatment – a therapy that equipped people with greater adaptability for life's other problems. Could modern therapy deliver more meaningful benefits to real people with more challenging difficulties? We shall see.

Post-CBT Therapy

As we have said, for more than two centuries physicians studied the pathology of the body and separated this from medicine of the mind. This division (or 'mind–body dualism'), which dates back to the age of the Enlightenment, has been described as Descartes' Error.[3] It is arguable who is to blame for it, but its folly is beyond doubt. Dividing the mind from the body is the biggest mistake ever made in the history of healthcare.

In reality there is no division between the 'mind' and the 'body', and so the historical notion of bodily 'dualism' is a myth. The truth is we humans are whole beings and our physiology is integrated. Illness experiences cannot be divided one from another. It is a mistake to say that such an illness is a physical illness and this other one is 'mental'. It is more correct to say, 'There is no health without mental health'; in practice, we know that poor physical health is the greatest source of premature mortality for those with enduring mental health disorders.

All modern therapies strive to be holistic and they all celebrate the value of a healthy mind in a healthy body. They respond equally to distress of the mind and to distress in the body, and through recovery they seek to unite the two in restored wellness.

The 'mind' in this new therapeutic context includes a wide range of human faculties, not only cognitive and behavioural ones. Modern therapies are concerned with more than thinking and behaving. Their concerns are emotional and interpersonal and much more besides. Human mental health problems are diverse; the real mental difficulties faced by people every day go beyond any single set

[3] A. Damasio, *Descartes' Error: Emotion, Reason and the Human Brain*, Vintage, 2006.

of experiences or problems. Modern therapists understand this reality and so they seek to achieve a more holistic recovery.

This is why none of CBT's established goals (behavioural and cognitive change) has been discarded by modern therapists. As we shall see, the post-CBT generation of therapists (such as Christopher Fairburn, Paul Gilbert and Marsha Linehan) made progress by holding on to the proven measurable values of Behaviour Therapy and Cognitive Behavioural Therapy. Their modern therapies refined established methods and then applied them to a more expanded human set of problems. The integration with BT and CBT therapeutic methods is a cardinal feature, but as we shall see later the modern therapists also harked back to more ancient sources of enlightenment, including mindfulness and the wisdom of older meditative traditions.

Mindfulness

The concept of mindfulness is one of the most helpful and hopeful developments of the modern therapeutic era. It is now so popular that it has become an established part of the everyday conversation about our mental health. So what is mindfulness? Why has it become such a buzz word?

The truth is that mindfulness means many different things to many different people. At one level mindfulness is simply a state of mind, an awareness of the present moment. At another level mindfulness relates to a technique of meditation, typically based on a focused appreciation of our breathing. The value of meditation as a tool for mental wellbeing has been recognized for centuries and across many cultures. Meditation in Buddhist, Hindu and Christian monastic traditions is part of an ancient set of wisdom, a wisdom far older than modern mental healthcare. So this mindfulness is the practice of purposefully paying attention to the moment in a non-judgemental way. Its exercise is sometimes referred to as 'practising being', tuning in to each moment in an effort to remain aware from one moment to the next. Mindfulness practice includes learning how to make time for ourselves, learning to slow down, and to nurture calmness and self-acceptance. Mindfulness allows the body to come to rest in the moment, regardless of whatever is on our mind or how we feel.

This mindful practice is said to promote awareness, empowering people to cultivate a kinder, more compassionate self. Mindfulness enables the appreciation of living in what its greatest exponent, Jon Kabat-Zinn, described as life in 'full catastrophic reality'. Not surprisingly this more mindful reality is a much healthier place to be. When we are mindful, our experiences become more engaged, more opportune and less fearful.

The benefits of mindfulness are enhanced when combined with a Cognitive Behavioural Therapy.[4] My focus on mindfulness in this book comes from this combined perspective. Mindfulness and mindful meditation are core skills incorporated into many of the new therapies described here. For example, as we shall see Acceptance and Commitment Therapy (ACT) and Compassion Focused Therapy (CFT) both teach mindfulness as a central tool. The sense of dynamism and enhanced consciousness brought to these therapies through mindfulness is one of the most important reasons for their success.

The 'Here and Now'

All the modern therapies included in this book have a 'here and now' focus. Like the behavioural and cognitive therapies that preceded them, modern therapies concentrate on the present and so they emphasize the potential benefit of a 'mindful recovery'. This mindfulness also allows modern holistic therapies to acknowledge a more narrative awareness. This is an awareness that focuses on acceptance of the present while simultaneously emphasizing the need for change in the future. Modern therapies aim to help men and women to reconcile such apparent

---

[4] The best source of information about this mindfulness-based CBT therapy is to be found in *Mindfulness: A Practical Guide to Finding Peace in a Frantic World* by Mark Williams and Danny Penman. The foreword is by Jon Kabat-Zinn, the originator of the mindfulness movement.

contradictions (for example, between on the one hand an acceptance of reality and on the other a commitment to change). This type of contradiction can be especially challenging. Nevertheless, as we shall see later, acknowledgement of such challenges opens up a whole new set of avenues for modern therapy.

Much of the scientific evidence supporting the effectiveness of mindfulness has been reviewed recently.[5] On the one hand large meta-analyses of clinical trials confirm the value of its use in treatment of depression and anxiety. On the other hand it is difficult to come to definitive conclusions about mindfulness. We still need to learn just how mindfulness works and for whom it should be used. This much is true: all modern therapies aim to be more mindful, more focused, more agile and more flexible. In this way they help people in their search for emotional peace and recovery. So are modern therapies really a route to a better life? We shall see.

[5] M. Farias and B. Delmonte, 'What is mindfulness-based therapy good for?', www.thelancet.com/psychiatry, Vol. 3(11), Nov. 2016, pp. 1012–13.

4

Paths to Wellness

ALL THE PATHS TO wellness described in this book are examples of more modern forms of therapy, but what is modern therapy actually like? I am often asked this question and the fact that I am still being asked it tells me at least one thing: therapy is still an unknown for many people. This 'unknown' has become part of the problem. People simply don't know what to expect when they see a psychiatrist or a psychologist, and the delay in seeking help arises partly from this fear of the unknown. So what can I say?

Each of the therapies in this book is included to illustrate some progressive and hopeful aspect of modern therapy. My intention is to show how holistic, humane and mindful mental healthcare works in the clinic. In reality modern therapy is a combination of these insights, used in an eclectic therapeutic mix, but for what it's worth I have separated these therapies in a certain order. This is simply to illustrate a progression, as I see it, from one therapeutic idea to the next. This order is in part a projection of my own, but hopefully it will work to illustrate the point.

It is said that the practice of medicine is an art. If that is so, then in my view medicine is an art made from a clinical craft. In mental healthcare that craft is psychotherapy. Like any other clinical skill psychotherapy is best performed when it is informed by both science and experience. Saying all of this still leaves the description of therapy a little barren, so let me go on a little further.

In an attempt to illustrate therapy perhaps it is best for me to reveal aspects of my own therapeutic approach. These may not be standard or universal. They are personal, even idiosyncratic, and they have been acquired over time. Maybe they say as much about me as they do about therapy, but they may also be indicative of real therapeutic benefit.

For example, my therapeutic practice relies heavily on metaphors and similes. I like to use poems and songs to illustrate the route to recovery and to encourage people to take it. For me, poetry and music fit well with therapy. They provide me with sources of language and illuminate the therapeutic relationship – the relationship between the patient and the therapist.

Of course each clinician will use their own vocabulary and each therapist must adapt this appropriately for each man or woman they work with. There is no single definitive lexicon of therapy, but, whatever the language used, a therapeutic relation-ship is always enriched by engaging conversation, warm dialogue and a plentiful source of meaningful imagery. In my view it's always best to see healthcare delivery in terms of a particular kind of relationship, the therapeutic relationship. That is why communi-cation is so vital.

This emphasis on communication may seem surprising. Some compare mental healthcare (either favourably or unfavourably) to systems of justice or politics, sport or theatre, or even to the circus. But if you were to ask me to compare therapy to something else, I would compare it to making music. Doing therapy is like making music *with* someone else. Of course this therapy could be like any kind of music, but for what it's worth the form of music I like to compare my therapy with is jazz.

This comparison with jazz music allows me to illustrate some-thing universal about all therapies. On the one hand each therapy is highly structured, and its aims and interventions are still very well defined. But on the other each therapy is new and each clinical response is adapted to an individual person and to a particular set of circumstances. It's a bit like jazz. Every jazz piece is defined and reproducible, yet each performance is unique and particular at the same time. Good therapy is like that. It's structured and yet new and individual each time, and that is what makes every experience of therapy so interesting and unique.

But still modern therapy remains a mystery to many people. Despite our fascination with the secret workings of the mind, we still have very little reliable information about the actual practice of therapy in mental healthcare. I like to quote the late Professor Anthony Clare as he used to say to me: 'The problem is that no one sees therapy *as it happens*.' Perhaps that is why it has remained a mystery for so long.

Unfortunately, as long as therapy remains a mystery stigma about seeking mental healthcare will also remain. That is why I am so keen to increase awareness of these new therapies and to show them to as many people as possible.

A More Multidisciplinary Approach?

Mental health treatment has changed immensely in the last thirty years. As we have said, there are now many new therapies and measurable ways of helping people to recover. Their focus has moved away from reliance on single modes of treatment such as medication or older talking treatments. Modern therapy involves more combined approaches and these are delivered along more plural multidisciplinary and focused paths. This broader, more flexible approach attempts to offer people greater access to different professional skills and to many other givers of care.

Modern recovery is best achieved with the support of this multidisciplinary team – a group of professionals working together to facilitate a recovery. This team includes inputs from nursing, psychology, medicine, occupational therapy, social work and other allied disciplines. Integration of all these resources at different times is essential. Hopefully the breadth of team membership helps to reduce the professional mystery surrounding mental healthcare. Each member of the team has a clear role, to contribute to the formation of a dignified and effective plan of care. So what then is a care plan?

What Is a Care Plan?

A care plan combines insights derived from the whole team working with each man or woman in distress. The modern care plan should be evidence-based, integrated and mindful of the rights and wishes of each individual patient. In the end a holistic way forward needs to be agreed. This is not always easy and conflict can arise, and as we shall see it frequently does, but through these challenges a respect for human rights remains the guiding principle of any care plan.

The team's recommendations are included in the care plan. These are based upon engagement with the patient as well as training, experience, research and hopefully common sense! When all of these things come together, a holistic and humane approach to recovery emerges. No thing and no one works alone. Human recovery prospers with mutual cooperation. There is a lesson in this: recovery can be hard work, so it is best shared. That's what team work is all about.

Of course, the nature of this 'work sharing' is what really matters. At the start of any therapeutic journey, it is perfectly natural to be apprehensive. After all, who knows what to expect? None of us can say exactly what will unfold in therapy. It can seem like a journey into the unknown. Sometimes people expect? the worst: the prospect of 'tea and sympathy' contrasts with the dreaded vision of the 'emotional boot camp'. Thankfully neither of these stereotypes will be included in our agreed care plans.

A More Mindful Recovery? The Potential for Modern Therapy

Simple solutions can seem attractive. We may be impressed by didactic advice and for a time we may find clear direction reassuring, but when it comes to mental health problems there are no easy answers – and no guarantees. A mindful recovery will not come from handed-down insight or well-meant advice. A more genuine mental health education is vital. Ignorance is not bliss.

As we shall see later, the route to mindful recovery is only made possible by a less judgemental and kinder experience of the present. This is the atmosphere of modern therapy. Mindful recovery requires us to harness time, helping us to live, to work and to love in each present new day. The experience of psychological pain is typically amplified by a kind of 'time warp'. This may actually be characteristic. Painful experiences are magnified by a lens that looks opaquely on the present and experiences only the past. As a result the stress we experience in the present is multiplied by the sadness and abuse we have suffered before. It is as if pain had wandered through time and space and chosen to visit us now. It brings with it all the painful afflictions of another time, another place and even another being.

For all these reasons modern therapies seek to resolve mental distress by rewarding clinical engagement in the present and building mindful therapeutic relationships for the future. Along the way they encourage restorative capacities like acceptance and commitment, courage and compassion, and most of all kindness. As a result they provide a more effective therapeutic menu, hopefully leading to a whole new plan for living.

Engagement with the process of therapy empowers recovery. Education about therapy is more meaningful when it involves personal learning and more than just an identification of past wrongs or a listing of targets for the future. Mindful recovery requires learning about the present, in particular learning about how to continue living within it. This learning about recovery is more practical and personal and tangible than people ever imagine.

New skills for living can be learned but acquiring new living skills requires a willingness to engage in therapy. This means experiencing therapy in an authentic, mindful way, with a willingness to acknowledge every challenge, even those things we find difficult to acknowledge, so as to learn from them all and hopefully move forward.

No one else can fully define the answers to our therapeutic questions. Each person in pursuit of recovery becomes the final author of a unique and personal diary of wellbeing. Every journey has some key moments and some truths with a universal quality to them. These epiphanies are not unique. They include experiences that are common to us all and so they too can be shared. These are felt particularly whenever we become mentally distressed or unwell. We shall hear some of these insights described later by my patients, but throughout each of these stories it is essential that we hold on to two objective realities: the first is that stress is universal in life; the second is that whenever we think we have reached the outer limits of our capacity we must be sustained by hope if we are to succeed. Even as grief, trauma and abuse bring with them great pain, they do not inevitably bring despair. When we triumph, it is by continuing. As the poet Robert Frost put it, 'The best way out is always through.'

PART II

Stories of Therapy, Recovery and Hope

THERAPY IS ALL ABOUT a special kind of conversation. That is why this book is built around a number of therapeutic conversations with my patients. These histories are composites of real care experiences, where each person's narrative is anonymized and the context altered so as to respect individual patient confidentiality. That said, my recollection of these conversations is as real as I can make it. Wherever possible, my patients have read and confirmed these pieces for their authenticity.

Each chapter includes a story in the context of a particular problem, a behaviour, a dilemma or an emotion, and each is an exploration of a modern post-CBT psychotherapy. Commentary on mental healthcare very rarely contains any good news, but, contrary to the prevailing pessimism, recent developments tell us that there are more reasons for hope than despair. Too little is said about the progress made in mental healthcare and in particular the many advances in modern post-CBT psychotherapies.

The choice of each of these new therapies is based on my own perspective as well as that of my patients. Recovery is a collaborative process of engagement. As you shall see there are frequent digressions as we talk, as in any conversation, and many potential paths are omitted. Therapy is, after all, about 'the road less travelled', to paraphrase Robert Frost again. The description of each process is naturalistic; that is to say it closely mirrors my experience of working with many men and women who experience mental distress and it follows their journey through the therapeutic process. The selection of modern therapies is also from my personal experience. My list includes the following:

- Enhanced Cognitive Behavioural Therapy for Eating Disorders (CBT-E) for Tara
- Acceptance and Commitment Therapy (ACT) for Laura
- Community Reinforcement and Family Training (CRAFT) for Robert and Barbara
- Compassion Focused Therapy (CFT) for Arthur
- Dialectical Behaviour Therapy (DBT) for Patricia

In the final conversation we will meet Joseph, as we witness a mindful consideration of integrated multidisciplinary care necessary for someone with a combination of physical and psychological problems.

My hope is that this book will be seen as an invitation to join in a wider conversation about our mental health and about therapy and our collective search for wellness. This is surely one of the most helpful and hopeful conversations we could have. You will appreciate that there are no easy answers here, but perhaps some of these questions might prompt or renew a dialogue, and that could be the beginning of a recovery.

Modern psychotherapies have much to tell us about the pursuit of a well-lived life. These new therapies are mindful and effective pathways to wellness, so it is essential that we do what we can to ensure these new treatments are made available to everyone who needs them.

Tara

TARA WORKS FOR AN IT company. She looks much younger than her twenty-nine years, but she is very overweight. Her GP asked me to see Tara urgently because she had been expressing 'suicidal feelings and a general loss of hope'. In recent weeks Tara had tried to end her life by taking an overdose of sleeping tablets. Her GP wrote that Tara 'is tormented with ugly thoughts about her body and her shape and her weight'. He wrote that she had been depressed, hopeless and isolated for many months. Tara, he said, 'was sceptical about her chances of achieving wellness with or without professional help'. He wondered whether Tara might have an eating disorder, or a problem with anxiety and depression, or perhaps all three.

In reality Tara was a young woman who had lost almost all belief in the pursuit of wellness. She had a number of coexisting serious problems and she had made numerous previous failed attempts at recovery. However, up till now for Tara the response to her problems had been fragmented and unsatisfactory. This much was clear. Rediscovery of Tara's health and wellness would require an entirely new approach to her problems and possible solutions.

When the GP's referral letter came to my team, we read it, as is always the case, at our regular multidisciplinary team meeting. This is a coming together of many health professionals, working as a team, and it involves a confidential discussion of the way forward for each person referred to us. After some consideration, the team came to the conclusion that in order to be successful this time Tara needed a combined response involving both medicine and psychotherapy. For Tara's care plan, the medical role and the therapy role would be shared between myself

71

and my colleague Pat, a skilled nurse and psychotherapist.

The form of therapy we chose was CBT-E (Enhanced Cognitive Behavioural Therapy for Eating Disorders), which is a specific and very effective therapy for patients with eating disorders. So what is CBT-E?

Enhanced Cognitive Behavioural Therapy for Eating Disorders (CBT-E)

CBT-E is a focused form of Cognitive Behavioural Therapy designed to respond to the particular mindset of someone with an eating disorder. This mindset includes the characteristic over-valuation of shape and weight. The therapy is focused on the specific thoughts and behaviours which maintain the eating disorder, but CBT-E ultimately uses this focus to influence many other aspects of an individual's life, from work to socializing and also relationships. To do this effectively it is necessary to start CBT-E by focusing on a small number of issues and resolving them first.

According to its primary developer Professor Christopher Fairburn of Oxford University, CBT-E is a powerful way of helping people with eating disorders to make changes in the way they think and behave. CBT-E encourages participants to analyse the implications of these changes in their behaviour and thinking as therapy progresses. The enhancement of CBT described by Fairburn and his colleagues refers to its focus on eating disorders and the specific nature of the individual therapy.

My colleague Pat had been specifically trained in this form of therapy and so she would guide Tara through its well-defined and detailed steps. Pat would see Tara regularly and together they would design the bespoke learning tools and exercises that she would need. My role was to support Tara and Pat by maintaining this focus and by ensuring the best possible care for her mood and anxiety.

Tara's Initial Assessment

Tara agreed to come to an initial assessment meeting where we talked together at length about her problems, her hopes for recovery and her wishes for a better life. It was at this meeting that we first spoke about the importance of her depression and anxiety. We agreed that these problems would need to be addressed together so that CBT-E therapy could succeed. Our assessment revealed that Tara had moderate to severe levels of depression with panic anxiety and so it seemed that Tara's mood would also benefit from some medication. We discussed the use of medication at some length and I carefully explained the risks and side effects. We agreed that, on balance, the potential benefits outweighed the hazards. Tara agreed to take an initial course of a medication known as a serotonin re-uptake inhibitor.

Tara and I also talked about her CBT-E. She was surprised to learn that CBT-E is effective for people with many different types of eating problem, including people with obesity or binge-pattern overeating. It is also effective for those with weight restriction (anorexia nervosa), and bingeing and purging (bulimia nervosa). Eating disorders come in many different forms, but most people with eating disorders share a similar problem: the overvaluation of weight and shape. The exact diagnostic description is not what matters most to CBT-E, it is instead the need for complete engagement with the learning therapy.

In CBT-E the path to recovery is about much more than simply matching a diagnosis and a therapy to a particular patient. A care plan needs to include a recognition of the whole person and this involves looking beyond diagnoses. This is why a multidisciplinary approach is so helpful. In Tara's story, as we shall see, it became clear that dieting alone would not cure her eating disorder any more than medication alone would resolve her depression. The combination of insights is part of the enhancement of the CBT therapy.

Tara's Journey Begins

Tuesday, 4 November 2014

It has been a few weeks since meeting Tara and during that time she has begun her CBT-E therapy with Pat. I am hoping to find out if Tara has clicked with the therapy and is feeling positive about it.

'Tara, it's good to see you again. How are things going with your therapy?'

'Not too bad now. Of course I was frightened about it at first.'

'Frightened – of what?'

'Ah, I didn't want to do the big "therapy" thing again. Raking through my past. I've gone down that road before. I've done the searching for nightmares, the walking through the horrible things said and done. I don't see much point in that. Why ask me to relive all that, and in the next breath ask me to just move on?'

'But the past has relevance, hasn't it? Don't you think the past is important?'

'I know you think the past is important. But I'm starting to see that it's actually done and dusted. It's over. Don't get me wrong, I am not despairing now and I'm not saying that the past isn't important, what I'm saying is that I'm more interested in the future. And the present.'

'That's great. It's really positive. But childhood is still worth thinking about when it comes to being well, isn't it?'

'Sure, but I didn't have a particularly miserable time in my childhood. No worse than anybody else. All you guys go on and on about it, but I don't see the point in fixating on it. Childhood is important, but it is not all-or-nothing. Anyway, that's the way I am choosing to see it this time around.'

'So therapy is making a difference this time?'

'Yes, it is. I feel like something's clicked. I'm getting on great with Pat. We're doing CBT-E.'

'And it's working well for you?'

'It's beginning to. We're looking at the old patterns. I'm finding new ways to look at familiar things.'

'Like what?'

'Like my body, of course. I can't ignore it. I mean, for years I have been looking at my shape and my weight. Too much, for sure. Checking all the time. I always feel like I need to be in control.'

'And what does "control" feel like?'

'Hungry! Fecking starving!'

'Well, that can't have been easy.'

'No, it wasn't. It still isn't. First I'd starve and be good and take control. And then I just couldn't take it any more. I'd break out and binge. I'd starve and then I'd binge. And then I'd do the shaming.'

'And what did "the shaming" look like?'

'Not pretty.'

'And is that when you would feel worst?'

'Sure, the whole thing became an exhausting ordeal. I would just retreat and starve and eat. Always on my own.'

'Why was that?'

'I wolf my food. I can't bear to let others see me eating.'

'And did you ever think about vomiting or purging or over-exercising or anything like that?'

'No, that's not me. I just check and starve and binge and loathe and isolate myself. Starve, binge, loathe. I'm sure you know the drill. That's enough to keep me busy, don't you think?'

'That's one way to look at it! Does it help to laugh about it?'

'It's dark humour. But I might as well laugh. I suppose I am a bit happier now that I've got a regular pattern in my life.'

'And getting back that pattern has been part of the therapy?'

'Absolutely. I'm finding that CBT-E is very practical. I'm learning new things, I'm re-evaluating.'

'Can you give me an example?'

'I'm learning to value other new things. Things other than *control*. All my adult life I have being putting myself through extreme challenges. I'm only realizing that now.'

'Extreme challenges?'

'It's hard to explain. But this is what I have been figuring out with Pat. I'm seeing now that all of my adult life I've been wound up, thinking about my body shape and eating and exercise. I have all these rules. I have made up all these rules, for how I eat and so on, and I was signed up to them. But they became too much. I couldn't follow through.'

'You know, Tara, sometimes recovery is about breaking rules.'

'Not just breaking them. Getting shot of them!'

'Well, tell me about your rules.'

'Oh, I've got lots of them, loads of rules. I have rules for everything I do, not just what I eat, but where I eat, how much I eat.'

'Can you give me an example?'

'Oh, I don't know. It's difficult to talk about it, but . . . one example I gave Pat is like this. Every time I pass a mirror or a window I've got to check that my bum doesn't stick out.'

'And you're trying to break that rule now?'

'Yes. Although I still look in the mirror, I don't punish myself based on what I see.'

'That sounds like the way to go.'

'Yeah, I used to look in the mirror and if I was unhappy I'd be miserable and I'd make myself not eat for hours and hours. I thought it was helpful, but it's not really. It's impossible to keep that up. I mean, clearly loads of women can manage it, but I know I can't.'

'Who manages it?'

'Oh, you see them all over the place. Stick insects on the red carpet. The ones in your magazines out there in the waiting room. No escape.'

'Do they make you feel angry?'

'I don't know if I'm angry. That might be a bit much. I mean, there's no point in being angry. But I haven't made this stuff up, this body stuff. It's everywhere.'

'I guess it is.'

'Oh, by the way, no mirrors.'

'No mirrors?'

'Yeah, you've no mirrors anywhere here. Well, you've one in the Ladies. I had to go in there to check myself. Like I said, this body stuff is everywhere.'

'Getting back to you, it's not just about being "fat" or "thin", is it?'

'No, that's right. It's about me, whoever that is. It's about me – not my curves.'

'And it's about valuing your real self, valuing you.'

'I guess.'

'Is that difficult?'

'Yes.'

'What feels difficult about it?'

'It means I have to give up my rules. And I hate that.'

'Why? What happens if you give up your rules?'

'If I give up my rules, I feel lost.'

Tuesday, 2 December 2014

It has been a month since our last session and I am interested to find out if Tara feels there has been a change in her relationship with food.

'Pat tells me that you had a session two weeks ago. How did that go?'

'Well, I'm learning about the process. I think I'm beginning to understand what I have to do.'

'It's great that you are working on all of this, Tara. Tell me, how are you putting CBT-E into practice?'

'Well, my eating at work is a big thing. You know I never used to let anyone see me eating, so I didn't eat at all. Not until I was home in the evenings.'

'And you must have been starving by then.'

'You bet. I could *really* have eaten a horse. Now I can see that I'm better able to work if I eat. Regular meals are good. And I am trying to eat with other people, not on my own.'

'This is good progress, Tara. And were you able to look at other aspects of your relationship with eating with Pat?'

'Sure, but for now it's regular meals, no postponing food. Pat says that's enough for now. It's all part of what she calls our "collaboration".'

'So you're taking one thing at a time?'

'Yes. The big issue for me was my mood, and I am getting a handle on that for the first time ever.'

'Explain that to me, Tara.'

'Well, I used to go like a yo-yo – from my eating issues back to my anxiety and depression. Back and forth. And that isn't happening now.'

'So you're able to concentrate with Pat on the "eating problem"?'

'On my *control* problem more like.'

Tuesday, 6 January 2015

Since our last session, Tara has met with Pat and I am hoping to learn how her care plan has evolved.

'How was Christmas for you, Tara?'

'It was quiet. But as you would expect there's a lot of focus on eating – and overeating – at Christmas. I could have done with having Pat in the house! There were times when I found it very difficult. I had to maintain control – not binge – whilst still being able to enjoy myself.'

'And do you feel you've made any progress since we last met?'

'I think I have, yes. I've clicked with Pat – and with you. That's part of it. I feel better after my sessions. I feel that each time we meet we move things along a bit – positive steps forward.'

'That's good. Maybe you can give me an example?'

'I'm trying to learn better habits. We agreed that from now on I would weigh myself just once a week. Only once! That's a massive change in my world.'

'Sounds good. And what other good habits are you learning?'

'Well, I am eating regularly now, whether I'm hungry or not. I never miss a mealtime. It's all planned out. And I don't leave long gaps between meals. Pat and I agreed times on all of that.'

'So Pat is mapping all this out for you?'

'I wouldn't say she's mapping it out *for* me. She's mapping it out *with* me. It's a collaboration. A team thing.'

'I see. So we're all in this together?'

'Yeah, I feel like she's on my team and so are you. For the first time, I'm really clear on my recovery plan. At least on paper.'

'Describe the plan to me.'

'It's lots of different things. For starters, we've a detailed diary that I keep. That helps me to monitor my eating. Pat told me that this would help me to understand the links between my eating and my feelings.'

'Looks to me like it would be a way of monitoring all of your progress.'

'Yeah, it is. We look through the records every week. I used to dread the weighing, but I actually look forward to it now. It's one of my favourite parts of each session because I can usually see that I have made progress.'

'And you'll keep going with the plan?'

'Sure. If it's working, why not? Pat's always saying: "The stuff that gets you well is the stuff that keeps you well."'

'Yes, that's right. We depend on that.'

Tuesday, 10 February 2015

Tara returns, having seen Pat. They have now established the weighing routine.

'The weighing can be dreadful. I always feel so exposed. There is no escaping the scales. I always used to judge myself by their measure.'

'Aren't you happy that you are seeing results, Tara?'

'It's not all about getting me thin, though. It's a little more than that.'

'What is it, then?'

'Well, when I used to weigh myself all the time I would feel miserable about it. Like my mirror-gazing and staring at my bum . . . I just kept doing it over and over, obsessively. Now I do it less often, only once a week, and I can rely on the result.'

'So that must free you up a good bit, leave room for other things?'

'Yes – in theory. But it turns out other things are hard.'

'Yeah. And they're linked, aren't they? Our feelings and the stuff we do.'

'I'm learning that. I'm trying to learn that. But it's so hard. It's not just about stopping the body-checking and the starving and bingeing and weighing. Pat and I have been talking about what she calls my toxic behaviours. I feel like I've a lot of those.'

'Checking yourself and avoiding eating in public aren't your only toxic behaviours?'

'No, I'm realizing they are more about isolation from every-body. This stuff keeps me cut off.'

'The body-checking and all the rest . . . wouldn't you love to lose those things?'

'I'm trying to do that. But I keep going back to them. They drive me mad, and I know they're not helping, but at the same time they're like my very own support system. It's hard not to go back to my old stuff.'

'Tara, how do you feel about all of us telling you what to do?'

'Well, it's not like I feel I'm going back to school or anything. But it is all so new. I feel you probably don't understand how new this has been to me. This is all new stuff that I have to learn. It has been very hard for me – and you guys probably take that for granted.'

'I didn't mean it that way. Just how do you feel about learning?'

'I'm happy to be learning. And I'm really trying. At least I think I am. It's just that I've never spoken about my mind and my emotions before. I don't know many people who do that.'

'I do.'

'I'm talking about *normal* people – not *psychiatrists*.'

'OK. Is that the way you see it?'

'Yeah, people don't go on like this in the real world. You know, the stigma thing is a big issue for me, and I'm sure it is for most people. No one wants to be classed as mentally ill.'

'Stigma?'

'We don't talk. And we don't talk about our *not* talking. Not in my world anyway.'

'But you know you can talk here, don't you?'

'Sure. I can do that because I'm being encouraged to express myself and I've never been told off by any of you.'

'Told off? Why would we do that?'

'I've had therapy before and it always seems like "do this, do that". This seems more . . . I don't know. But it's like you and Pat have given me permission to talk about myself and how I feel, and whatever I say I know you won't tell me off. Like I said, these aren't the conversations you have in the real world – or not in my real world!'

Tuesday, 4 August 2015

Tara dropped out of therapy for many months. When she returns, she looks downcast. Her weight has gone up again and when we meet she seems frustrated and angry.

'Tara, how have you been?'

'Well, I'm back here again, so . . .'

'It's been six months, hasn't it? Why has it been so long?'

'Lots of reasons . . . I don't know. Maybe my life just got in the way.'

'It's good to see you again. You know that, don't you?'

'I'm not so sure!'

'Seriously, it is. But why has it taken so long?'

'I suppose you could say I have been in a crisis.'

'Crisis?'

'I thought I was so much better, like I had it all figured out, but I realize now that I haven't. Now I just feel really stuck. It's a terrible feeling.'

'Everyone feels stuck at some time. What's it like for you when you are stuck, Tara?'

'All my plans – for getting well – they're all confused in my head. I can't remember where to focus my attention. And all the concentration on my eating behaviour, as you guys call it, seemed to miss the point.'

'How?'

'You seemed to leave me out – me, Tara – who I am. I was left totally out of the picture.'

'Oh Tara, no one here wants to leave you out of the picture. Forgive me. Is that what we did?'

'Yeah, it sort of is. But I'm not looking for apologies. From where I'm sitting, my problems are mine and they are more than just difficulties with eating. If I just needed to focus on that, I could have gone back to my local fat club. I mean, if that was all there was to it.'

'But there is more to it all than just being overweight, Tara?'

'Of course, I understand that. Don't you remember why I came here in the beginning?'

'Sure I do. It was because you were so close to despair. And as I remember your anxiety and depression had become too much for you.'

'And do you not remember, at our last session – it didn't go so well, did it?'

'Didn't it?'

'I felt we were going nowhere fast. Look, you gave me the plan on paper. So, like, once the plan was set, all I had to do was follow it. But doing it is another thing.'

'You're right there. It is.'

'And it seemed to me that all of my real problems were forgotten.'

'Forgotten? By who?'

'By you and Pat. So it felt like all I could do was go back to doing what I know best.'

'You mean the body-checking and bingeing and avoiding people?'

'Yes, all of that.'

'But things can be different, surely?'

'But I don't see it. I don't see how. Pat always said I was unique, so why do I have to change so much? There is all this focus on my eating and the plan. I just don't feel like me any more. I mean, I can follow the guidelines, if that's what you want . . . but it just leaves me wondering, you know?'

'Wondering?'

'Well, for one thing, what am I doing coming to see you? Why don't I just go and talk to Pat? She's always so helpful to me. I'm wondering why am I here, why am I seeing you?'

'Tara, please, let me tell you how things seem to me and why we can both be very hopeful. You're right, your problems are not straightforward, but actually nobody's problems are. Sometimes recovery is like a house of cards. If we pull a card away – any card – the whole house falls down. So if we were to stop working on any of it, on your mood, or your anxiety, or your eating, then the whole recovery plan might fall down.'

'But isn't that what I'm saying? I wanted you to sort out my other problems too, not just bang on about my eating issues. You sent me off to Pat and somehow everything else just got lost.'

'Sorry, Tara, but that's not the way it seems to me. And it's certainly not what we ever intended. Pat and I are working together and we are a team, your team. The way we see it, all of these issues are linked and so none has priority and none can be avoided.'

'I don't know. I really just don't understand where we're going with all of this.'

'Tara, your recovery is our only priority. And that's about the whole of you, not just one or other of the issues. We're not going to pick and choose here. It's good you have come back. That's what is so important. And it is so hopeful. We can pick up where we left off.'

'But my anxiety is back and my weight is up. After all this time, my bloody weight is up! I felt like I couldn't go on some of the time. I couldn't do all of those things all of the time. You were asking me to spin plates like I was some kind of a circus act. I'm not a magician. I get confused and upset and then I'm back to square one – feeling bad, and looking bad . . .'

'Just hear me out, Tara. From our point of view, getting well is about continuing. So your recovery is all about keeping on. Being well is about keeping going. And so there is no point in saying: *Because I'm not making progress in this area or that area I'm going to stop working on my recovery altogether.*'

'But that's not what I'm saying. I want to get well. I want to do this. I want to be well.'

'Well, that's great. We know you can be well. And look, you came back. That's what you've done. You're the one bringing all the issues together. And that's what we're here for – you and Pat and me – working together as a team. Your recovery is about bringing all these things together, doing lots of things at the same time and yet trying to focus on doing some of them really well.'

'But I felt like we failed at that last time. I couldn't do everything at once. And we didn't exactly pull it off.'

'Maybe. But that's OK. You came back, that's what matters. And it shows you have the desire to try again. Together we will manage your mood and your anxiety as well as your eating. None of these things is a reason to despair or to abandon the work on your recovery, Tara.'

'Well then, if that's the case you need to know that I stopped the medications. I just felt, I don't know, to hell with these tablets! I know there's no shortcut to getting well, but I kept thinking, why do I have to take these? Other people don't have to take tablets every day.'

'So, what are you going to do?'

'Well, now I'm here I guess the question is, what do you advise?'

'Tara, it's a question of doing what works for you. They were working well. Your anxiety really reduced, and your thoughts and mood became so much better. You were getting on with Pat and doing the CBT-E. My memory is that we reviewed this often and it was very clear that you were doing well. But it's not an issue of right or wrong.'

'What do you mean?'

'I mean that no one is telling you what you should or shouldn't do. It's whatever works for your recovery. Let's give it another try.'

'It's that simple?'

'It can be. Why complicate it? After all, feeling better will give you the space to deal with the other things in your life.'

'Well, I just wish I was feeling better and had a bit of head space. Sometimes I just have such a sense of shame. It's awful. I know there's still a fair bit of work to be done on my eating and judging myself. But there's more to it than that, isn't there?'

'There is. Our emotions are not so easy to re-learn.'

'You spoke about "surfing the urge" when I wanted to binge and snack. I'd distract myself and go for a brisk walk – I mean, even I can't stuff my face and walk at the same time – and from that, well, the urges just kind of passed for a time. Can you "surf" your feelings as well? I mean, how do I change feelings and emotions that I have lived with all my life – how do I re-learn those? Sometimes I don't understand any of this, not at all. I just thought that if I did my homework this time things would be much better.'

'Well, perhaps it is easier to understand if I put it like this: getting well is about more than just learning to manage your weight and your eating. Together we can learn to change other things as well. Your thoughts and your feelings can change.'

'So I guess I'm taking on more here than I did at slimming club?'

'There's a lot more to this learning, and I know that coming here takes a lot out of you. But getting well is not just about improved time-management or reorganizing your diary so that you keep your appointments. Actually you're really good at organizing stuff already, Tara.'

'But I'm not managing well. I've gone back to my old way of doing things. Last week was awful. I got a wedding invitation and it has put me into a total spin! I immediately felt desperate and so scared.'

'I'm sorry to hear that. Tell me, who's getting married?'

'My friend, Kate. We were in college together and we worked together for years. She's lovely, but she's asked me to do a reading. Can you imagine – me, up there in front of everyone?'

'You're well able to do that.'

'No, I'm not. I'm really not! Don't you see? If I do it, I'm going to be out there on show. Everyone will see me up there. I've started looking in the mirror again, checking myself constantly.'

'And how do you feel about that?'

'A failure, of course! What else can you call it? As I said, it's shame. I'm back to square one again. I am obviously a failure. For one thing, I'm not slim.'

'That's not the only issue, is it?'

'Perhaps not for you, but I thought at least I'd learned not to look in the mirror. Not to care about this stuff any more.'

'But you do care.'

'Yeah, I do care, even though I thought I was shot of this. Maybe I just can't do this. I feel very anxious again.'

'Everyone goes back before they go forward. This stuff isn't easy.'

'No, it's not.'

'But look, you've come back. So you're happy to see Pat as well, aren't you?'

'Do you think she'd see me again, after all this time?'

'Of course she will. Would you like me to talk with her?'

'Would you?'

'Absolutely, Tara. As we say, whatever works.'

Tuesday, 25 August 2015

Tara comes back to therapy, having spoken with Pat about the reasons for stopping. She still has many questions, but she is beginning to look at things in a broader way.

'So, your session with Pat went well, then?'

'Yeah, we talked about everything really. About why I stopped coming, and about starting again, and she said much the same as you, that she would be happy to start back. We're going back to CBT-E.'

'Great, so where did that take you?'

'Lots of the old stuff, but some new things. For one thing, we did a pie chart. I never thought that pies would be part of my solution!'

'Well, like we always say, you've got to keep an open mind.'

'Seriously, I was shocked by that pie chart. Seeing things in black and white like that, it really scared me. We used it to zoom out and look at the bigger picture.'

'How did that look?'

'Shocking, really. We were looking at my life and dividing things up according to where I put my attention and how I judge myself.'

'And what do you pay attention to?'

'The truth is a very big slice of the pie is for shape and weight.'

'And there's not much room left for anything else?'

'That's right. There has never been much room for anything else. But I know that needs to change. I need to get back my focus.'

'And how might it change?'

'I'd like to see other things in that chart. I need to make the shape and weight slice much smaller.'

'And how might you do that?'

'Pat says it's by making other slices bigger.'

'Like what?'

'Like . . . things I enjoy, for example. There's lots of things. I like to travel and meet new friends and maybe, who knows, even have a relationship. You know . . . things everyone wants.'

'So, Tara, where would you start?'

'I'd like a slice for dancing. I'd like to be OK going to this dreaded wedding! I need to have more in my head than my shape and weight.'

'You're absolutely right. I'm so pleased you're seeing it this way.'

'It's going to take time, isn't it?'

'Of course. It does for everyone. But tell me, how is your mood and anxiety? You seem a little more contented.'

'My anxiety is still there, but it's not as much of an issue.'

'So is depression on the pie chart?'

'My mood is an issue, but it's a smaller piece of the pie.'

'So are the other pieces more about your life as a whole?'

'Yes, they are about me, not just what I think. I suppose that's always been a part of the problem.'

'Go on.'

'Pat said I was going to get here at some point, where we would be talking about other things.'

'And it's not just dancing, is it?'

'But that would help, wouldn't it?'

Tuesday, 22 September 2015

Tara has become fascinated by the treatment and sees it as positive that she is being encouraged to eat.

'You know I have done ordinary CBT before, but it didn't work.'

'But this is working for you now, Tara?'

'This time it's different. Pat seems to know everything about my eating problems.'

'And about how to help them?'

'Of course. That's why I'm here. I'm not interested in wasting any more of my time. It's like this time I am learning so much more. It feels like we're learning together. And, you know, it's the weirdest thing but Pat actually wants me to eat. That surprised me at first. Pat says I can eat – so long as I eat every four hours and stop my long starve times.'

'So Pat's given you a meal plan?'

'Yeah, breakfast, lunch, mid-afternoon snack, evening meal and even a snack at night. Who would believe it? I feel like I am eating more than I ever did!'

'Or maybe more often, more regularly?'

'Yeah, I get it. Of course you know I'm a binge eater, never did other stuff like purging myself or throwing up or using laxatives – yeuch! I just binged. So now I am not allowed to give in to the urge to eat at other times. We have come up with lots of what Pat calls good "distraction activities" – same as before, like going for a walk or phoning a friend or even having a shower at those times when I am dying to eat.'

'So you're keeping busy!'

'So busy! But it's a good kind of busy, and it's helping me make progress. I am really learning to surf my urge!'

'You like that turn of phrase?'

'Yeah, it's like a new language I'm learning. A healthy language. I used to talk about "calories" all the time, but now Pat says we can talk about "energy" instead. It's somehow less distressing. For me *calories* are bad but *energy* is good.'

'It's a whole different perspective really, isn't it?'

'Oh, definitely. And CBT-E is very detailed. I mean, my meal times are set down in the plan, there is no more of my eating from packets or off the frying pan. I used to pick at food between meals. Basically I'd be nibbling all day.'

'What does Pat say about that?'

'She calls it grazing! Now I don't do that. I am also trying to eat more slowly – that's a struggle – and I try never to eat while I am watching TV or doing other stuff. Pat says from now on I am to eat "mindfully". "Savouring one mouthful to the next."'

'Non-judgementally?'

'Yeah, that's a laugh! But I am getting there. I used to be so critical of everything and every part of me.'

'Yes, wouldn't it be great to be less hard on yourself?'

'I have made progress there. For one thing, I don't feel full all the time now. I used to feel that way – especially after a binge. It's an awful feeling, like when you have eaten too much and your body is about to burst. It's like feeling your clothes are too tight and you just feel fat.'

'Tell me, Tara. What's the connection between feeling full and wearing tight clothes and getting better?'

'You must understand, it's about the ways that I judge myself. Thinking about my body size and shape and weight makes me sick of myself.'

'What do you do when you feel that way now?'

'I try to remember that it's not all about me. Don't get me wrong, I am not there yet, but I know now that people can't see my tummy sticking out, so I don't have to wear tight-fitting clothes or stuff that is just too small for me. It's what Pat says about judging myself by my shape and weight. No one else is judging me, so why should I?'

'If only we could replace all this judgement with respect – more respect for ourselves.'

'Pat says the type of respect we need is more kindness. That's it in a nutshell, isn't it?'

'Yes, kindness to yourself. It is the beginning of recovery – and it's our end.'

Tuesday, 13 October 2015

I notice a change in Tara's behaviour. She seems more confident than on previous meetings and more relaxed.

'So, now you have a tattoo?'

'No, no, I said I'm *thinking* of getting one. And I was wondering what you thought of that.'

'Lots of people get tattoos. They are very fashionable. What's important is what you think about it.'

'It's about my focus. Pat says that what you focus on grows. So maybe if I can put all my body focus into a single tattoo I can leave it out there for others to see. I could let the focus on the rest of my body go.'

'And would everybody see this tattoo?'

'Maybe, but actually I don't need my tattoo to be like a huge scar. I am not replacing my body consciousness with something else, but maybe it's something I'd be happy to show off sometimes, when I want to. It won't be seen every day in the office.'

'What would it look like? What would it be?'

'I don't mind. Maybe something small and beautiful on my shoulder.'

'And the wedding?'

'Well, I think I'm definitely going now.'

'Are you ready?'

'I've got to get the dress and I would love to get fit. My weight is coming down but I still want to be in good shape physically.'

'And psychologically?'

'Of course, I am happier now. My shape and weight aren't the only things. I have learned that. I remember I was so miserable when I first came here.'

'Yes, back then you felt so low in yourself.'

'It was just the thought that there was no way out. That was the worst.'

'But now things are very different?'

'Yes, I have been seeing Pat regularly. She says moderate exercise is good and so I am trying to go out more. I am running now! Who would have thought I would say that?'

'We did!'

'Maybe. But now Pat says it's time to take stock and begin designing the rest of my treatment.'

'And you're up for that?'

'Yes, more than ever before.'

Tuesday, 17 November 2015

I am looking forward to seeing Tara. I know it is coming towards the end of her therapy and I am wondering how she is going to incorporate the therapy into her day-to-day life.

'So, I suppose you want to hear about the wedding?'

'Of course. Tell me all about it, Tara.'

'It wasn't a fairy tale or anything, but it wasn't a disaster either. I'm really glad I went. For Kate, for my friend. She was so happy I came. I've kind of been backing out of things like that in recent years.'

'And you did the reading, did you?'

'Yeah, I did. And I had the *frock*. That was the most interesting bit.'

'Why?'

'Well, you know I put a lot of thought into the dress. The style, colour, sleeves or no sleeves, and I bought it thinking I might have that tattoo to show off. By the way, I didn't get the tattoo, not yet anyway. I still might some time. But I bought the dress – it was sleeveless and I felt good in it. Anyway, the most interesting thing was that there was another woman there and she was wearing the exact same dress as me. It was the weirdest thing.'

'How did that make you feel?'

'Actually, I was OK with it. Amazing!'

'What did you do?'

'I just went up and talked to her. We had a "snap" moment. Twins! Once, in the past, I might have freaked out about something like that, perhaps even run off. But this time I didn't – in fact, it was a bit funny. I knew her. I was at school with her sister, so later on when I bumped into her in the Ladies we both just laughed about it.'

'So, in a way you met your double?'

'I suppose. Sort of.'

'And how did the rest of the day go for you? Did you enjoy it?'

'Somehow I just wasn't as concerned about how I looked as I used to be, so I was able to enjoy the day. I was even able to take a Ferrero Rocher off the tree and eat it. Imagine me, eating in public – that is impressive!'

'Good for you, Tara. So, where do we go from here?'

'I've been talking with Pat about ending the therapy. It's been very much on the agenda in recent weeks.'

'But that's a good agenda, isn't it?'

'It is.'

'You've made so much progress with the way you feel about yourself. Look at how much you've achieved. You do feel better, don't you?'

'Yes, I do. And now I know that the stuff I was doing to myself before was no friend to me.'

'I'd like to think you really believe that.'

'I do. It's just that the stuff I've been doing – self-loathing and starving and bingeing. I'd been doing it for so long.'

'Ending your therapy doesn't have to be sudden or final. The door's always open, if you need to come back.'

'But, you know, at this stage I'd really like to move on.'

'Absolutely. There's so much more for you to do. And so much more for you to feel.'

'For the first time, I'm glad about that. I'm less frightened. Can I say I'm looking forward to it? Is it too wild for me to look forward?'

'No, not at all. Let's look forward. Now that you are happier in the present, you can look forward. It's great to look forward.'

'I'm really grateful to Pat. I feel the CBT-E she introduced me to has made such a difference.'

'Yes, it is hard to find people like her. It's one of our biggest challenges.'

'But there's something else I want you to know, Jim. Getting better . . . it's not just about Pat and you. Something changed for me when I came back in August.'

'What was that?'

'I think it was just that, you know, I was *ready*. I needed that time and space to make positive decisions, and that was important.'

'And you're ready now?'

'I am.'

Tara's Journey

Tara's CBT-E used many of the techniques associated with BT and CBT and added just a little bit more. According to Chris Fairburn, eating disorders and CBT are perfectly suited to each other.

Tara's CBT-E helped her to reframe errors of thinking typically associated with eating disorders and it did this by using an extended focus going beyond limited diagnostic categories. CBT-E is a modern therapy. It is egalitarian, practical and measurable. It acts directly within the everyday practicalities of a person's life. For example, Tara gained a different perspective by looking at the pie chart and understood a great deal about her behaviour by keeping a diary of meals and emotions. There is nothing obscure or esoteric about it. It's about learning.

Today, Tara is doing well. She has a new job and a new set of plans for the future. She still sees Pat, but only intermittently. Tara's binge-eating, body-checking and anxious avoidance have all been reduced. And now if she judges herself, or her past or her future, that judgement is less through the prism of her weight and shape. She has been enlightened by new understandings gained through her therapy and her subsequent recovery.

Shame was a recurring emotional theme for Tara. She felt shamed by others and ashamed of herself because of her shape and her weight. Body-shaming, as it has been called, is not a new phenomenon, but it has become more alarming in our age of social media. Through therapy Tara found that we had no room for shame and so in time neither did she.

Tara needed to exchange the negative image of her body shape and weight for a new personal, less judgemental image of herself. To do this, she needed first to feel better and then to behave in different ways. Through focused CBT-E she was able to make substantial changes in her thinking about herself and in her behaviour around food. These cognitive and behavioural changes were her first substantial gains.

Tara's mood and anxiety also improved and so, in many ways too, Tara felt well. Her multidisciplinary path to progress allowed her to engage with every aspect of her recovery and so to make real changes to her way of life.

Tara's journey taught me many things. Listening to Tara reminded me that more complex problems require more focus and take more time; both things were accomplished through CBT-E. In Tara's case, the problems of binge-eating and obesity were complicated by anxiety and depression. Returning to CBT-E therapy after dropping out for a time was a significant breakthrough. There was a sense in which Tara's hopes for her future were reignited by her return. She began to believe in the possibility of a life beyond bingeing and extreme body consciousness. Even still, nothing in Tara's life has been determined and who knows how she will live it. Her potential was restored and that is what matters.

Overcoming avoidance behaviour can be difficult. When her therapy began, Tara was afraid. Seeking wellness was hard for her. It is still too hard for many people. Tara once said that only psychiatrists – not 'normal people' – talk about their minds and their emotions. Tara reminded me that stigma surrounding mental health remains our biggest obstacle to recovery.

Persisting with therapy can also be hard. Even when we think we are making progress the job of putting these steps into practice may be just a stretch too far. Tara's decision to break from therapy, and more importantly her decision to return to it, were the determining events in her recovery journey. The specifics of CBT-E were important, but even more so was Tara's renewed engagement with the CBT-E process in the long run.

Mental health problems can be all-consuming. When we are not well, our emotional energy is drained and so we cope by using avoidance and by reducing the scope of our life. We turn to 'safety' behaviours that at first seem to us comforting. We stick to these behaviours because we think that they will help us, but as we have seen with Tara avoidance behaviours eventually become a more toxic support system than we ever intend them to be. In truth, avoidance behaviours give temporary relief but at a very high price.

Just as Tara was on the brink of recovery, she faced the greatest dilemma of her life and she had a choice to make. She could move towards wellness, with all its unknowns, or she could stay with what she already knew, the thoughts and behaviours she had been stuck in for so long. Happily Tara actively re-engaged with the process and she was able to take it a step further. It was then that we both discovered how much we had misunderstood one another. Her return gave us all – Tara, Pat and myself – a welcome chance to try again.

Why some people engage with therapy and others don't may not be fully understood. We now know that many factors play their part in this engagement process. For me, the availability of therapy, as well as awareness of its effectiveness, must have something to do with it. There is a need for more trained therapists (such as Pat) and for greater access to effective therapies such as CBT-E for eating disorders. Our first job is to let more people know that help is available. Our next challenge will be to deliver these effective therapies to everyone who needs them.

Tara reminds us that even with the best will in the world recovery may take many attempts, but that's OK. What matters is that we work together for wellness and that we keep trying.

Laura

LAURA IS A SIXTY-TWO-YEAR-OLD married woman with a past history of depression and anxiety. Laura had not been to our clinic for many years and so her return was unexpected. Her GP sent me a very brief referral letter suggesting a review was critical. All it said was that Laura was in the middle of 'a personal crisis'. Her GP gave no further details, except to say that she felt 'the matter was urgent' and that now she was 'worried for Laura's safety'.

When someone is re-referred in this way, it is best to review the previous records. These may not always be easily located. Data protection legislation requires that old notes are kept on file for up to twenty years after the last clinical contact with mental health-care – after two decades following last contact all records must be destroyed and by right.

Even though it was a long time since I had seen Laura, her file was still available. It confirmed that she had an address in Dublin. She was married to Tony and he worked for a bank. Laura and Tony had one son whose name was John. Before she married, Laura had worked for a time in a legal office and then for some years as a flight attendant. She had retired after John's birth and (at the time of our last meeting) she not been employed since.

Laura's first episode of depression had occurred many years previously following John's birth, but it appeared Laura had made a full recovery. She had followed up with me on a number of occasions for similar episodes and ultimately she had returned to the care of her family doctor. Nothing in Laura's notes gave me any clue as to the nature of the crisis.

Laura's Initial Assessment

When we meet, Laura is abrupt, impatient and emphatic. We chat for a few moments before Laura reveals the reason for her referral. She has become involved in buying a benzodiazepine sedative online and is now addicted to the drug. She expresses her feelings of shame and desperation at having been caught. A recent delivery in the post has been intercepted by Customs and Excise, the outcome of this being that her dependence on Valium is no longer secret and she has been forced to face the reality of her addiction.

Our meeting is an opportunity to create a care plan whereby we can approach her addiction with compassion, however Laura finds it hard to see an alternative future. When I tell Laura that I will not prescribe the drug for her and that rather we should look at other options for recovery, Laura is initially hostile and frightened, but soon her defences are lowered and her feelings of hopelessness and anxiety are revealed.

I suggest a detox as a first step, which she will approach with the support of her GP, then I recommend Acceptance and Commitment Therapy (ACT). This modern therapy is ideal for people who feel 'stuck' in their lives and who struggle to manage their thoughts and emotions effectively. Its process of 'acceptance' has helped many patients with anxiety disorders and addictions to benefit from this empowering psychological intervention. It is a very positive step when Laura agrees to think about accepting help.

Acceptance and Commitment Therapy (ACT)

Acceptance and Commitment Therapy (ACT) is a modern behavioural therapy developed in 2005 that encourages 'psychological flexibility'. It does this in a number of ways by teaching people mindfulness skills and by enabling men and women in distress to reconnect with those things that matter to them most – their true values. ACT aims to realign the actions of an individual with their values. In this way ACT helps to move people closer to where they really want to be.

ACT therapy can be delivered in groups or in one-to-one sessions, but it is particularly appropriate wherever psychological rigidity has become an impediment to recovery for people who feel 'stuck'. ACT builds on the methods of CBT, but it differs in a number of important ways. It does not view difficult feelings or painful emotions as 'errors' in need of correction; instead, ACT teaches us to remain *present* with the difficulties of life and so instead to move closer towards other more valued thoughts and behaviours.

To this end, ACT makes great use of mindfulness: helping people to live more in the moment, connected more to what matters, and making the most of each and every day. These mindfulness skills can help us to unhook our feelings from unhelpful thoughts.

The ability to look at things from a fresh perspective is a real strength, adding greatly to our mental health and wellness. ACT teaches this by promoting six specific skills, which are mindful connection, thought diffusion, expansion, values, perspective taking and committed action.

1. *Mindful connection* is the ability to live more mindfully in the moment.
2. *Thought diffusion* is the ability to 'unhook' ourselves from unhelpful thoughts.
3. *Expansion* refers to the ability to overcome uncomfortable and unwanted emotions.
4. *Values* are those thoughts and beliefs that are most important to us. According to ACT, a realignment of ourselves with these true values is restorative.
5. *Perspective taking* means learning to connect more with our observing self. That is the part that takes notice without excessive judgement and so manages to see a bigger picture. ACT encourages the ability to review things from multiple different vantage points.
6. *Committed action* is the ability to do today whatever it takes to be well. ACT teaches us to break down our long-term goals into smaller pieces, then take action by taking smaller steps in

sequence towards those goals. By teaching these skills ACT helps us to get back on track.

The experience of ACT shows that psychological flexibility can be learned. This flexibility is an essentially resilient capacity, one that allows men and women to adapt their point of view, to become more accommodating, more present, more conscious and, in the process, more mindful. In times of mental difficulty psychological flexibility helps us to re-focus our behaviours on our real values. With this renewed 'values-driven' mindset, a recovery can grow, sustained by new thoughts and renewed hope, anticipating new experiences and new joys.

Laura's Journey Begins

Thursday, 29 October 2015

After our initial meeting, Laura decides to meet the team. She has started her detox with her GP, so I am interested to learn how things are going.

'Tell me, Laura, how has your detox been going?'

'I won't lie to you, Jim. It's been tough. No two ways about it. My GP is still giving me some sleeping tablets because I begged her for something – but obviously the drugs are not working. At this stage I am going to need something more than a good anaesthetist!'

'Well, there are other ways of making progress. I am really keen on you doing ACT, Laura.'

'I know you are, so I did speak with someone in your team about it.'

'Julie?'

'That's right, Julie. She told me lots about it. She was very nice, but even still you know I'm a sceptic about this sort of stuff.'

'Part of the idea of ACT, Laura, is to develop an open mind, a more flexible approach.'

'Easier said than done, but I do want to feel well. I'm not sure I deserve to be happy, but I don't believe we were all put on this earth to be miserable. I think all that "valley of tears" thing is pure crap. But Julie said something to me that shook me.'

'What was that?'

'She said my mental health has to be about more than just knocking me out!'

'She's right about that.'

'She asked me what I really cared about. About what she called "my real values" and, you know, I just didn't have the words to answer her.'

'What is holding you back?'

'I don't know. Fear? Shame? Stigma? I don't know what it is. But I can see that it's choking me. I have tried everything else.'

'What do you mean?'

'I must have read every self-help book under the sun. I know all the advice: "be fitter, happier, more productive". Give me a bloody break! I have struggled for years, trying to do something about this. I am just stuck. Sometimes I wonder if I know who I am at all.'

'Do you want to talk about that?'

'Of course! I wouldn't be here if I didn't have things to talk about.'

'So let's talk about ACT. You've spoken to Julie, our ACT facilitator. She is a psychologist. It would be great if you could go to Julie's ACT group. Once you've got through your detox, the ACT group could really help you make a fresh start. What do you say, Laura?'

'This time, Jim, things have to be different.'

'This time they can be.'

Tuesday, 17 November 2015

Despite her scepticism, Laura completes her detox plan in consultation with the team. This meeting is to review her progress and hopefully encourage her to keep working with ACT.

'My GP says I am depressed, but somehow I know there is more to it than that.'

'Like what?'

'I am anxious all the time. "Depression" is such a catch-all phrase, isn't it? Seems everybody is depressed nowadays.'

'Are they?'

'Yeah. Everyone's got a "diagnosis" of some kind. Even in showbiz. You can't get a platform unless you've a diagnosis. This guy's depressed. This girl's bipolar. It seems to be almost fashionable to have some kind of depressive illness!'

'Sometimes, Laura, terms like depression are just words. They don't necessarily tell us much about how we actually feel, still less about what we do.'

'Now you're sounding like Julie in the ACT group.'

'How are you finding the ACT group?'

'Look, Jim, it's early days, but I am trying to give it a go. She teaches something she calls "diffusion and expansion". Julie keeps telling us that we can learn to see things differently, from different perspectives.'

'What kind of perspective?'

'That's it, Jim. Maybe I am just too depressed.'

'Is that what you really think?'

'No, I'm not saying I'm actually depressed. What I really feel is that I'm anxious.'

'Anxious?'

'And it's not some silly superstition either, but I have to live within my boundaries, my safe places. I won't walk under ladders. I even count magpies. I know that sounds trivial – though I suppose it's quite common – but my fears are not trivial. I'm frightened and anxious all the time, and everywhere I go. And I'm frightened about everything I do.'

'And is that why you avoid as much as you do?'

'What else can I do? I have been avoiding everything and everyone for years. I use Valium to live and now you won't give me that any more. Neither will my GP.'

'Laura, can you tell me more about your anxiety?'

'It's hard to talk about it.'

'Try to describe it for me.'

'I don't like to think about it. It's like a . . . background tension. When it stays with me, it paralyses me.'

'And do you ever get crescendos of anxiety, panic attacks, where your heart beats so fast you think that just maybe you are going to die?'

'No, not now. That's where the benzos came in, Jim!'

'Apart from taking medications, what else have you tried?'

'I've dipped in and out of a few therapies, but never for very long. I used to go to reiki and aromatherapy. And I did a bit of a mindfulness course, once.'

'And did any of those work well for you?'

'Eh, not really. I tried to go with all the whale music and the hot stones. But I've gotta tell you, for me the benzos worked better. Here's the thing: I just can't handle anxiety and pain. I don't want my life to be such a struggle.'

'And has it been a struggle, Laura?'

'Look, I have to work hard at things. I'm good with my diet. I take care of my body. I stay in shape. And I run. That makes me feel good, but it's not that extraordinary. So much has happened in my life and none of it is extraordinary.'

'Will you tell me about your life, the ordinary and the extraordinary? Tell me about who you are.'

'I will have to think about that.'

Tuesday, 15 December 2015

Laura has decided to engage with the ACT group and has been introduced to mindfulness.

'I am going to the ACT group and it is helping me. Julie says the plan is to meet about eight or ten times in total. I was a little apprehensive about joining her group, but I am going along with it.'

'How many people are in the ACT group?'

'There's eight of us and they are a nice bunch. Julie insists on confidentiality. It's part of what she calls the "group agreement". Disclosure, she calls it "sharing", is going to be hard for me, Jim. We spent a long time discussing trust at the first meeting.'

'It takes time, Laura, but what else have you been doing in the ACT group?'

'There's been a lot of stuff about mindfulness, but somehow it's different from before. Now I realize mindfulness can mean lots of things to lots of people.'

'Are you finding it more relevant now?'

'It's got all the usual ideas. You know, about living each day moment by moment, non-judgementally, but now I can see that Julie is trying to get me to consider my whole life less judge-mentally. Seeing the bigger picture. She calls this "perspective taking".'

'That makes sense, doesn't it?'

'Maybe it does, to you, but it seems a contradiction to me. It's hard to understand how living moment by moment can be done while taking in a bigger perspective at the same time.'

'Hmm, that takes real flexibility, doesn't it?'

'You bet it does. I am definitely not there yet and, anyway, my thinking is always so unhelpful. I don't like to do much thinking about things. My style is to keep things firmly locked in Pandora's box. I never give any room for that sort of thinking. Thinking about my life just makes me feel so uncomfortable.'

'Do you ever talk in the group about that?'

'Like I said, I have never talked before.'

'I know, but maybe this time you can have a changed conversation.'

'It's all just words and they just say the same things all the time.'

'Laura, words don't have to be the same. Why don't we start talking about what you really care about, about your life and your values? Maybe we could look back a little. We could talk about the things that used to matter.'

'Julie says I need a new language, but that's not easy to find. My natural way is very straightforward.'

'It's not all or nothing, Laura.'

'Maybe so. I remember back when I was flying – first we were called *air hostesses*. A few years later they brought men in – they were called *air stewards*. Later they called us all *flight attendants*. What did it matter?'

'Pot-ay-to, pot-ah-to.'

'Tom-ay-to, tom-ah-to. You said it! Words! Do you know that when I look back on my life I find it hard to recognize much of it now?'

'What's it like, looking back?'

'It's like I'm watching a play, and like somebody else is playing me. I'm not really there. Maybe I don't want to be there.'

Laura is restless at this point, as though she is struggling to tell her story. There is more for her to say.

'Sometimes, Laura, life is challenging because of what *hasn't* happened as much as because of what has.'

'But stuff has happened to me, Jim. Don't you see? I have a past.'

'We all do. The question is, what does it mean for you now?'

'I thought my past was all bad. I just wanted to blot it out. I find this hard to say, but living in the present isn't getting any easier. Tony, my husband, will soon be retiring. John, our son, is living away. Somehow life is not to be what it should be, not what it might have been.'

'Do you mind, Laura, that we talk here about these very personal things?'

'I suppose you would say I am at the stage where I have to talk about them. All I can say is that I'll do the best I can.'

Tuesday, 12 January 2016

Laura returns after some sessions with the ACT group. This time she is more earnest than ever before.

'How did the detox go for you, Laura?'

'Oh, it was the time of my life, Jim. A laugh a minute . . . Actually I hated it. Every day I wished you guys would just leave me alone and give me back my benzos. "Set me free", like you said. Hah!'

'Valium would have been easier, Laura, wouldn't it?'

'Which of us is the smart-arse today, Jim?'

'Irony is not what you're here for?'

'I don't know what I'm here for. You know I have tried straightforward mindfulness before and I know all the lingo. Like I say, to me it's just words. They have their meaning. I used to know what suited me. Now I feel desperately trapped and anxious all the time. I don't know if anything will work for me. Other people are probably more straightforward . . . I suppose it's my fault.'

'Why do you say that?'

'Look, I am just not a very psychological person. I see things more practically, more definitely as being this way or that way. I believe in right and wrong. Things are sometimes done the right way and other times the wrong way.'

'And when you think of your life, do you think of it in that black-and-white way?'

'I don't know how I think of life. I can't ponder my life. I don't know what an ideal life would look like actually.'

'Try to imagine it. Maybe you could picture it for yourself. Could you?'

'I don't do daydreaming, Jim. Waste of good time.'

'Laura, let's try. Let's do some imagining.'

'Are you serious?'

'Yes, let's try it. Come on. Think of it as a form of ACT, a diffusion of thoughts. I'm OK with that. Are you?'

'All right. It's a waste of your time. Since you're asking, I would say that in the past . . . I dreamt of travel, I wanted to have a career, but I gave all that up a very long time ago. Then, for a while, I hoped for a big family. All the trimmings. Maybe I just wanted to be kept busy. I suppose I just didn't have the courage in the end.'

'You're very hard on yourself, aren't you, Laura?'

'Maybe I am.'

'Have you ever considered how strong you have been?'

'Never. But sometimes Tony says that. Sometimes. I don't pay any heed.'

'Is Tony part of the life you dreamt about?'

'Well, he should be, shouldn't he? He is my husband after all!'

'Tell me about Tony.'

'What's there to know? Tony is quiet. You know, the silent type. We go about our lives. We were both lucky to have one child. No more came along. Back in those days we just accepted that. I was glad to have John and after my depression I knuckled down to raising him.'

'And what about John?'

'He's great. Never put a foot wrong. Takes after his dad in that way. But he's an easy-going lad. I suppose there are some advantages to being the only child.'

'Like what?'

'We gave him the best chances.'

'What age is John now?'

'Twenty-five. He left home last year. Moved to Italy with his girlfriend. To Tuscany. She's a nice girl. She was an au pair for our neighbours some years back. That's how they met. Apparently, her mother makes the best focaccia in the world. Johnnie loves Italy – and everything Italian.'

'How does that make you feel, Laura?'

'It's the way now, Jim. It's just that we see so much less of him. *I* see so much less of him. They say they are saving up for a deposit for a house. I think they're going to get married next year. I would love to think they would come back here, but who knows?'

'And Tony, how does he feel about John moving on?'

'Oh, Tony lets everything go. He's what the ACT group and Julie would probably call psychologically flexible! Actually "anything for a quiet life" is Tony's motto.'

'But you're different?'

'Yep, I suppose I am. We are a real yin and yang couple. Tony retired recently after nearly forty years in the bank. Forty years in the one bank! Can you imagine? That's my Tony.'

'And what do you think about a quiet life with Tony, Laura?'

'Truthfully, if I had my choice, if I was back in my youth, the old me, I would be looking out across the world. You know I used to fly . . .'

'I know you did. Transatlantic flights, that must have been exciting?'

'Hmm . . . maybe, in comparison to my life now. I suppose you think my life now is very ordinary, very boring.'

'Actually, Laura, not at all. That's not what I meant at all.'

'Sometimes I just don't know what you're thinking, Jim!'

Tuesday, 16 February 2016

Laura seems more relaxed and so she talks more freely, more openly, about her fears.

'My fear, Jim, is that without my Valium I will have no safety net. My anxiety will torment me.'

'Sometimes feeling distressed can be OK. After all, ACT is about acceptance. Do you feel that you're getting better at dealing with your distress?'

'Maybe mindfulness is working for me. I haven't had any panic attacks for a while, but if they were to come back I don't think I could cope.'

'So that's why you think you need the Valium, to avoid the panic?'

'Yes, of course. I needed something to dampen down the sense of stress and anxiety I felt constantly. Surely you can understand that?'

'No, Laura. Really, it's not as obvious as all that.'

'Yes, it is. To me, at least!'

'Benzos only lead to more avoidance – you can end up avoiding everything else as well.'

'For sure. But that's OK! Valium takes care of the lot.'

'But Laura, the Valium is in your past.'

'Not in my mind, but maybe it will be soon, Jim.'

'And so once your life is without Valium, what will your priority be?'

'I told you, I am not a woolly thinker. If I think about things, I only end up being the loser.'

'It's not about being a winner or a loser, Laura. You're off the Valium now. You're doing your mindfulness. You're participating in the group. You have done really well.'

'I am not there yet!'

'Have you talked about what matters for you in your ACT group therapy?'

'Others have shared far more with the group, but I'm not ready.'

'Maybe this would be a good time.'

'Jim, I have so many issues with this, I don't know where to begin.'

'It's not easy, but it's better to go for it.'

'Why do I need to talk to the group about any of this? I don't want to be part of some circus, some freak show!'

'You won't be, please don't worry. Of course you can talk more about this again, but for now would you feel able to give it a go with me?'

'Tell you? Regardless of how scary this is for me?'

'Yes, tell me *because* it's so scary.'

Tuesday, 15 March 2016

Laura returns and this time she is keen to talk. She is animated and intense.

'I have to tell you, I never want to go back there.'

'Where?'

'Back to where the panic is – back to the stress of it all.'

'So that's why everything has to be kept hidden, under lock and key? Your feelings just stay in that box?'

'Where they belong!'

'And will that make your fear go away?'

'The Valium would do that.'

'But it doesn't, not really, does it? You know all this avoidance of fears just makes them grow larger.'

'You keep saying that and it's easy for you to say, Jim, but I still want some peace. I don't need more hassle. I believe in moving on.'

'What does your version of "moving on" mean? It sounds to me more like "moving away"? And doesn't that come at a cost to you?'

'What cost?'

'Laura, it just seems to me that you have cut yourself off. Cutting yourself out of the picture. Imagine a dentist whose only remedy for cavities is to pull out every single tooth. Avoiding all anxiety means we avoid lots of things in our lives. In a sense this approach is just about making yourself immune to feeling. That's no way to live.'

Laura pauses briefly and turns to look out of the window. Then she begins to speak.

'When I was younger, I expected more from my life, but in the end I had to reduce my expectations. There was no other choice.'

'Talk to me, Laura, about the life you had before.'

'How long have you got?'

'Let's look at it together.'

'What do you want to know?'

'Tell me about your family.'

'We weren't particularly wealthy, but we weren't poor either. No one had money back then. My father was in the civil service. My mother was a housewife, a homemaker, whatever you call it, what does it matter?'

'Where did you come in your family?'

'There were five of us, so there was no money for piano lessons! And there was no money for me to go to college. The nuns told me I could be a nurse or a teacher – or even a nun, God forbid!'

'Why?'

'I was too fond of going to dances! I suppose I could have been a nurse maybe. I'm good at looking after other people.'

'Were you ambitious?'

'I couldn't wait to grow up and get away. One of my brothers went to the USA and he never looked back. But I met Tony and things just seemed to fall into place.'

'If you had it over, would you have chosen another career?'

'I would have liked to go to college. I was smart enough. But I did the usual secretarial course and got the usual office job.'

'Did you enjoy that?'

'At first I liked the freedom. I loved having my own money, even if it was only to buy stupid things. I loved being on the move: getting the bus into town and walking the last few streets to the office each morning and evening. There was a buzz in the city back then. I'd be giddy just going about my day. I found it hard to keep a straight face.'

'Office work suited you?'

'For a time, but I was never going to do it for the rest of my life. I didn't fit in. I think I was too outspoken for them.'

'So you decided to fly!'

'Up, up and away, Jim! Back then air travel seemed so glamorous. All the boys wanted to be pilots and all the girls wanted to be air hostesses. People would take a day trip out to the airport just to see us in our uniforms and watch us taking off around the world.'

'And you saw the world, didn't you?'

'I was on transatlantic with stopovers in New York. We were on the jumbo jets, so they called us the "jumbo babies". Actually I was never a "jumbo". But we were just babies – we'd lots to learn. It was damned hard work, but I was up for that. And some good things did come out of it, too.'

'Like what?'

'For one thing, I met Tony.'

'What was it about Tony that you liked?'

'The way he carried himself. So self-contained, a real cool

customer. Whenever I could manage it, I would bump him up to first class and we would talk.'

'It was a happy time?'

'Yes. For the most part. Until the incident.'

'What do you mean, *incident*? Can you talk to me about that?'

Laura pauses for a much longer time. As she continues to look out of the window, she speaks without returning my gaze.

'This is not easy. For me.'

'I know. None of this is easy. But it will be OK to talk about it. Trust me.'

'I have to tell someone about what I have been thinking.'

'We can talk. It's OK.'

'I don't think about *it* all the time. Some of the time my mind is a blank, but I never forget about it either. You can talk about your mindfulness, Jim, but my problem is that my mind is already *full*. It's full of all the wrong stuff. My mind is so full of this.'

'Laura, you can tell me about whatever is on your mind.'

'It's about something that happened back then, some "carry-on" in the hotel on one of our New York stopovers. I suppose it's just the usual ugly sort of thing that happens. I feel terrible even talking about it.'

'Laura, let's talk about it, even though we both know it feels terrible.'

Laura continues, almost without hearing my reassurances. She is weeping a little as she speaks.

'It happened late at night, on a two-day stopover. We were always so careful, trying to spot a dangerous situation or a dodgy character. The more experienced girls would make sure you kept your bedroom locked day and night.'

'You looked after each other then?'

'I suppose so. We really did. Occasionally we'd have these room parties. We would all go to one of the rooms and we'd bring a few bottles of wine, but this one time it got completely out of hand. By the end of the evening, I was feeling the worse for wear. I really just wanted to get back to my room. One of the senior crew said they'd bring me back. Maybe I gave her the wrong signals.'

'So, what happened?'

'We never called it rape – not back then – but I suppose that's what it was. Certainly she had sex with me and I didn't want it, if that's what rape means. I was a virgin. I wasn't married at that stage. How could I explain it? I didn't even have the words.'

'And now, when you think about it, what comes into your head?'

'I remember her bad breath. She stank of booze. And her perfume. I never forgot that. She never hesitated, even as I resisted her. And she was violent – no doubt about it. I was floored. She was one of the girls and I trusted her. I never saw the threat. We were just talking.'

'So what do you do when these memories come into your mind?'

'I don't let them come, if I can help it. I try not to think of it. I fight it whenever it comes into my mind. I am not even sure I want to be talking about this now. This is very distressing . . . Maybe you don't feel my story adds up to much, but this has been my life. This has been my life and it's all but ruined me . . .'

'I understand how you feel, and I know your feelings about this are real. What I am saying is that there is no denying this happened. It's just that fighting how you feel must be so hard, so emotionally exhausting.'

'I prefer not to talk about it. I do whatever it takes to make sure these things stay out of my head.'

'And still, Laura, these really unpleasant memories just come right into your head when you least expect them.'

'Yes, and I am left living with a kind of waking fear.'

'And that can't be easy.'

'I have a lot of shame. Somehow I feel I could have done more to prevent it or stop it. And I am on the lookout for hazards around every corner. I used to find the threats almost anywhere. Nowhere was safe. It was awful. Awful. Awful.'

Laura is wiping her tears now, struggling to continue.

'It's OK to cry, Laura. You're right, this is awful. But hopefully it's better that we have talked about this. In fact, it might be the best step – *because* you're distressed – that we talk about this.'

Laura is visibly upset.

'Would you like to do this now or another time?'

'Jim . . . I would like to stop talking now. This is too much for me. Can we take a break?'

'Of course, Laura. We can stop now.'

Tuesday, 19 April 2016

Laura has come to a turning point in her therapy, allowing herself to talk about her past. A big part of ACT is acceptance and so I am interested in Laura's thoughts on this, as her therapeutic journey continues.

'Last month's meeting was very painful. Laura, did you feel it made things worse to talk about it?'

'No, it didn't make it worse. You see actually I get the point. Better out than in, right? I've been avoiding this for so long.'

'It's all about "acceptance".'

'Acceptance? The ACT group talks a lot about that, but what the hell does it mean?'

'It means a lot of things. Acceptance is essential for all of us: for you and me.'

'This is the bit I don't get. Look, Jim, are you really trying to tell me that I have to accept being raped? Where do you get off? Try telling that one to the women of the world, Mr Psychiatrist, Sir!'

'No, Laura, that's not what I am saying.'

'That's what it sounds like to me. Acceptance, indeed. You mean that your much vaunted recovery is just about telling me to keep putting up with being violated? That's *un*acceptable! ACT group – great, huh?'

'*Your* ACT group, Laura.'

'Yeah, too right! What an ACT!'

'Laura, the acceptance we're talking about is the acceptance of how things make us feel. It's not about accepting what happened. It's not about putting up with rape or any other horrific crime. Real acceptance is about acknowledgement of the facts as well as the truth of your feelings. You're not wrong about any of this. Accepting your feelings means we don't have to deny them or put them in a box or blot them out with Valium!'

'Yeah, Jim, you always come back to that one, my Achilles heel, but look, Jim, I am the one who lives in the real world. Don't give me more wordplays. I am tired of it. I want to know what to do.'

'But, Laura, this ACT therapy could really work. We're not playing with words here. I know you think this stuff is mumbo-jumbo – just a lot of chit-chat – but let me try and explain. It's a really helpful idea, acceptance.'

'No, Jim. OK, I get it, but now you have to understand, I have never told anyone else before about what happened to me. I certainly haven't told Julie or my ACT group!'

'Oh, I see. But Laura, I'm not going to tell you what to do. Our only goal is your recovery. That's what we value. And recovery means change. We believe you can change your behaviour even though you have all of these painful feelings.'

'But supposing I don't want to make a change?'

'Change is going to come anyway. There's no future for any of us by avoiding change. The only question is how we handle it today – how can we learn to stop hiding from it?'

'But this is so hard for me.'

'Yes, and that's why it's really important that you don't lose hope.'

'But, Jim, what good will acceptance do for me?'

'Laura, with acceptance you could fly again.'

'Give me a break! It's flying got me into all this trouble in the first place, Jim.'

'Suppose what we mean by "flying" again is "living" again in a more present, more mindful way, living with your stress. Not avoiding it or feeling ashamed of it and needing to put it away.'

'Jim, I need things to be real. I don't want to pretend that things are better when they aren't. I may be going to the ACT group, but I am not acting – even if I can be quite a good actress, Jim! I guess I've had to be. But now I want something effective. I want to live. But my problem is I feel so anxious.'

'Laura, let's talk about that "but".'

'Excuse me? What did you say – talk about "but"?'

'Yes. *But.*'

'What about *but*?'

'That *but* could be an *and.*'

'*And?*'

'How about this, Laura? How about changing "I want to live *but* I feel anxious"? Let's change that to something more useful. How about this? I *will* live *and* I will feel anxious.'

'You mean I can feel anxious at the same time and not be overwhelmed by it? That would be something, wouldn't it? I think you might be on to something there, Jim.'

Tuesday, 10 May 2016

At this meeting Laura seems perplexed.

'Don't you understand? I always believed that I should never go back to that pain. I felt I had to get on, just get over it and be normal. Have a normal life. Be the wife and be the mother . . . It's the stigma, Jim. It's just huge for me. Huge.'

'Laura, we all feel it, and—'

'You know, Jim, I've been thinking a lot about Julie and my ACT group. We are coming up to our last session and I feel curiously guilty.'

'That's the last thing any of us want you to feel, Laura!'

'Well, now I am feeling it, so that's OK. Don't you say I have to accept what I feel?'

'That's true, but what makes you feel guilty? To my mind, you have nothing to be guilty about.'

'It seems to me, Jim, I have not been entirely honest with the ACT group. When we made our "group agreement" and we trusted each other to confidentiality, other people really shared, but I haven't. At least not yet.'

'And are you going to share now?'

'It won't be easy, but now I see it's the right thing to do. We have talked a lot about acceptance and now I am beginning to understand. More importantly now we are getting to do something about our issues. It's the phase Julie calls "committed action".'

'Yes, that's when the group talks about "doing whatever it takes to be well".'

'So Julie talks to us about breaking down our long-term goals into smaller, more do-able steps and taking them one by one, so that we get life back on track.'

'Maybe it is time, Laura, to start talking about your long-term goals?'

'But first I want to be honest with the group. I haven't ever told them about my rape. And that must mean my issues probably don't make any sense to them. Somehow I need to tell them now, so that we can plan the way ahead.'

'Laura, can I ask you another personal question? What do you value about your life, or more precisely where do you see your future?'

'Being with Tony. He retired recently, so for us it's a bit like starting again. He's a bit like my dad: long-suffering.'

'In what way?'

'There is so much I have never told him. He knows something about New York. I told him a version of it, but . . . but I've never been able to find the courage or the right words to explain to him just how awful it all was. As I said to you some time ago, it's because there's a part of me that feels I could have prevented it or stopped it, so I think there's a sense of guilt that hangs over me. And Tony is not someone who talks about feelings very much, so I had a good excuse to suppress all of this – to keep it locked away.

Looking back, perhaps the fact that he keeps things to himself is what attracted me to him.'

'Laura, would it help to talk more openly to Tony now? Maybe he would be willing to come to see me with you some time?'

'I don't know, but I can ask him.'

'It's your call, Laura, but if it would help, we can do it.'

Tuesday, 14 June 2016

Laura brings Tony to our meeting. Tony is a slim man, neatly dressed in tweed jacket, tie and suede shoes. He seems reticent at first, but he insists that he is happy to join us at our meeting. After Laura introduces him to me, Tony takes his seat and waits for a moment, as if he needs an invitation to speak.

'Tony, thank you for joining us today. Is there anything in particular you would like us to talk about?'

'Dr Lucey, Laura told me that I should address you as Jim, but I suppose she knows you better than I do. I am happy to call you Dr Lucey, if that's OK?'

'No problem.'

'I'm aware that Laura has been through a lot in her life – she's had to cope with many difficult problems – and sometimes I feel there's very little I can do to help her, which frustrates me. Now I'm very sad about what happened to Laura in New York and I find it upsetting to look back and realize we have never spoken about that. I'm a bit angry, I suppose, that it's taken us until now to talk about things. The first I knew about just how awful it had been for her was when she came home from here two weeks ago. Up until then I think we'd only touched on this.'

Laura interrupts at this point, as if to clarify what Tony is saying.

'It's been a tough few days, Jim, I can tell you. But I was determined to tell Tony everything – Julie said it would be better if it all came out.'

'Indeed, we sat up all night on Saturday. I haven't cried in years – believe me, Dr Lucey. But I cried that night. And I haven't been like that in years. I have lots of regrets.'

'Regrets about what, Tony?'

'I always thought Laura knew that I was her biggest fan. Perhaps I didn't say it enough. I admit I am not the most demonstrative person. But I regret that I never said enough before. I think the fact that I tend not to talk about emotions and feelings doesn't help things – I bottle them up – but Laura knows now that I will support her in every way I can.'

'So, how have things been for you and Laura since you retired, Tony? Have things been different?'

'Laura is more anxious. I know what she told you, but she was not always so anxious. Obviously, she had her episodes, but that's normal, isn't it?'

'You mean her depressive episodes?'

'Yes.'

'So in between the episodes, what was life like for you, Tony?'

'As I said, it may not be the impression Laura gives to you, Dr Lucey, but we have been happy. Overall, I would say we have been happy. It's not all meant to be plain sailing. But Laura and I have stayed together and we have raised our son. On the whole, I'd say we have had a happy life together. Certainly life has not always been this difficult.'

'When did you come to know about Laura's addiction, Tony?'

'I'm obviously shocked about it. I just had no idea. But I've always been proud of Laura as my wife.'

'What made you most proud, Tony?'

'My wife has always been a great help to me. In the early years of our marriage it helped us so much that Laura worked as an air hostess. I was just starting out with the bank and I admired Laura for her spirit and her hard work. I never heard about the New York episode – or at least I never realized. I just knew there was never anything glamorous about Laura's work, and it could be tiring and stressful – which is why I appreciated her doing it to help with our finances, as we started out together.'

'Tony used to say, Jim, that whereas *he* occasionally flew to the US, *we*, that's me and the other girls, we used to "walk the Atlantic" every week!'

'Yes, that's right, I did say that. Laura worked hard and I never resented her for retiring.'

'Explain that to me, Tony.'

'Well, Laura always made her choices and I accepted them, Dr Lucey.'

'Perhaps that's not quite the kind of "acceptance" we have been talking about.'

'Sorry, Dr Lucey, I have no idea what you're talking about.'

'Tony, now I must apologize to you. I should explain. Laura has been talking in ACT therapy about accepting the way she feels yet still living.'

'We did accept things. Once Laura's health went I didn't expect her to return to that life.'

'It's so interesting, Tony, that you use the word "accept" in this way. For us, it's an important word. It has many meanings. Laura and I have been doing a lot of work around the meaning of acceptance. Particularly around her addiction.'

'You don't need to give me the details of what you're doing, Dr Lucey.'

'I think it could be helpful, Tony. Do you agree, Laura? Do you mind if I share with Tony what we mean by "acceptance" in this room? You've been doing a lot of work around this, with the ACT group, are you happy for me to share this with Tony?'

'Go for it, Jim. I'll just listen if you want to explain the nuts and bolts of the therapy. Tony finds this mental stuff very hard, though. I suppose that's one of the things we have in common.'

'You know, Tony, when Laura and I talk about "acceptance", we are not asking anyone to accept the unacceptable. Our kind of acceptance is a generous action. It's one that we can take for ourselves. It allows us to own how we feel. It's not about putting up with intolerable things. But it can be about allowing us to do things even though they're painful for us. It's about getting going again. Acceptance helps all of us to move on in the present with our feelings.'

'I wonder sometimes, Jim, if Tony and I should have asked more of ourselves.'

'Is there another way of looking at that, Laura? Maybe acceptance is about making a life together now and still keeping that kind of question in your minds. What do you think about that, Tony? Do you think it would be worth exploring this line of thinking?'

'Maybe. In any case, I'm here. And like I said, I'm willing.'

Tuesday, 2 August 2016

Laura comes to see me some weeks later. Her manner is much more relaxed now and she seems brighter, fitter and more hopeful.

'I've made some changes. I'm trying to make great changes. And I've taken most of your advice . . . Actually, it's not all about your advice, that's all well and good. It's your encouragement, Jim, that really mattered.'

'Thank you. You've probably hit on something there, Laura. What we need is encouragement, not advice.'

'Yes, ACT helped me realize that I wanted to give up fighting my fears and my past. I started to think about it more. I didn't want to abandon it this time.'

'And Tony is playing his part, isn't he, Laura?'

'You know, Jim, he is a good man. He's talking more and he's listening more, and did I tell you we are doing mindfulness training together now?'

'And so things are improving for you both, together?'

'They are. We're learning to be together again. Warts and all, Jim!'

'Laura, you have come a long way since you detoxed.'

'I feel really well. I cannot tell you how much better I am. It's been ten months now.'

'That's fantastic, Laura.'

'The help I was offered before . . . I suppose I only took it partially. I saw things only one way. For better or worse – and mostly worse. I see now that there was an elephant in the room: my anxiety. In fairness, nothing could have worked for me while I was on the benzos. You were on the money there, Jim.'

'And Julie and the ACT group, did therapy make any difference for you?'

'ACT's been huge. For me, it's become a partnership like I would never have imagined. Some of the ideas that came from Julie and ACT have been totally new to me. Remember I had only done my version of mindfulness before. This time it was different . . . That's acceptance, too. And trying to look at things differently. It's been a big leap for me. And I like the idea of taking committed action. I am rediscovering my values and my goals. And now I am working towards them with Tony.'

'And how are you managing without the benzos?'

'It's still very hard but, as I said to Tony, *I may have craved, but I haven't caved!*'

'Good for you, Laura.'

'This time I'm trying to take my future in bite-size steps. That's important, I think. I needed to take it at my pace and stick with it. You know I wasn't convinced by the ACT stuff at the start, but actually it has really helped me. I want to push through.'

'I'm so glad about that, Laura. I accept this is difficult.'

'You're telling me! In fairness, though, we have had a few laughs along the way.'

'We have.'

'Remember when you told me that ACT was about learning to sit with difficult things? I have to tell to you, that made me laugh out loud!'

'Why, Laura?'

'Sit with difficult things – try sitting with Tony in traffic on your way to an ACT session! I'd rather walk the Atlantic any day!'

'But you are sitting it out, Laura.'

'I am, and I'm keeping going. So good riddance to the benzos! I guess you did set me free in the end.'

'Did I?'

'All right, I'm setting myself free.'

'You are. And what does "free" look like?'

'In a curious way that I hadn't understood before I am much more free without the benzos. Before this I used to be checking all the time that I had them near me – in the glove compartment of the car, in my handbag, at my bedside. I needed to see them so that I could feel safe. They were like good-luck charms – except, of course, they weren't good luck at all. I can't say they were bringing me much luck. I can't tell you how much of a prisoner I had become. I thought they were my crutch, but I know now that they were actually preventing me from owning the reality of my past and taking on the possibilities of my future.'

'That's a whole new ACT way of looking at things. Of course, it might be harder than you think to maintain your independence from the sedatives without help, Laura.'

'Well, it helps a lot that I've come to like you, Jim. Well – not like that, don't flatter yourself! No, I can see that I was sceptical at first. I dismissed much of what you were saying as mumbo-jumbo, just more of the bleedin' obvious.'

'Yes, you did, but it's OK to be sceptical. Those feelings are also real, so it's worth holding on to them as well. The important thing is that we keep moving towards recovery – *with* our feelings, not despite them.'

'I get it now, Jim. I really do. I guess that's what you meant about being free, being and feeling at the same time.'

'You know, Laura, you're not going to be a different person, but you can have a different life.'

'With the same feelings?'

'Sure, sometimes, but that's OK, isn't it?'

'I suppose so, but remember I'm still learning about mental health.'

'You and me both.'

'Yeah, it's not just the usual advice about exercise and diet and lifestyle. I nailed all that stuff a long time ago, Jim.'

'So what's different now, Laura?'

'Now I want to be open to possibilities. I'm trying to be open to new ways of minding my mind. I realize now that none of my old techniques – my meditation tapes or my reiki or my aromatherapy oils – could ever have worked for me, really.'

'Well, maybe we see it a bit differently, Laura. There are lots of ways of minding the mind that work. And those techniques could be good.'

'But not while I was on the benzos, right?'

'That's right, and not without acceptance of how you feel. And committed action for change.'

'I'm trying to get that acceptance. I'm thinking a lot about my difficulty with changing things, Jim.'

'Like what things?'

'Well, like the stuff you said about seeing things only one way. Do you realize that I couldn't see the wood for the trees before?'

'In what sense?'

'I had tunnel vision, I think: I could only see the bad stuff. Don't get me wrong, I still see all the bad stuff in life. There is plenty of it around. But I'm starting to see the good stuff at the same time.'

'Sometimes it's hard to see the good things that are going on all around us all of the time.'

'I'm starting to recognize that. And I'm learning that not everybody feels happy all the time – and many of us have had to learn to live with traumatic events. That was huge for me. And knowing too that it's not actually *mad* to have negative thoughts and anxieties and feelings.'

'We all have negative thoughts and anxieties, Laura.'

'And I can't force them out any better than you can. I'm learning that. I'd try to force them out from time to time, sure, but then I'd come across something that would be too strong to force out and I'd feel like I'd lost the battle, then I'd reach for the benzos. And I know that's just a dead end.'

'There's lots there to think about, Laura, isn't there?'

'Of course there is. Even the small things. I've always known that eating well is vital. Goodness knows that was drummed into us when we were the jumbo babies. You know they used to actually weigh us?'

'Really?'

'Yes, every month one of our managers used to line us up and weigh us on a set of big scales. Of course she never flew, that's for sure. As far as I could see she just filled out forms and weighed us.'

'Imagine how different things were back then.'

'Yeah, and there was no fear of her fitting into one of those pencil skirts!'

'That's a bit harsh, Laura, isn't it? Don't you think so?'

'Why? Can't I be angry now? I've told you before, Jim, I'm no hippie. And you told me before, you're not going to ask me to accept the unacceptable. This manager seemed to take pleasure in humiliating us.'

'You're absolutely right. That must have been a horrid ordeal, and some of the other things you have told me about and have had to endure were terrible. They did happen.'

'And yet now you're going to tell me that since they're over I must get over them?'

'No, they're over, but other good stuff has happened as well. Your life story did not stop at that moment, at that moment of violation. Other stuff happened and most of it has been good and life progressed and so your life was not stuck on an angry note.'

'Look, Jim, I'm trying to get it. Julie said there was a difference between having anger and having an angry life.'

There is a pause in our conversation at this point and it seems as though it has reached a tipping point. Laura is still struggling with the apparent contradictions in her feelings. Despite much progress it is still hard for her to identify the best way forward.

'We're having a lot of these pauses today, Jim. Meaningful moments, are they called?'

'But that's OK, Laura. Reflection can be good. An angry person doesn't pause.'

'True. But you have to remember I am still the same person, so

I guess the question for me is this: What now? What next?'

'What do you want to do, Laura?'

'What I'd like to do is spend more time with Tony. Having him back has been a big part of all of this "getting well" thing.'

'Having Tony back?'

'Well, having him here. We've decided we're going to do a whole lot more together. We'll go to the mindfulness classes and we're learning how to manage our stresses. He is very sympathetic, really. And we have already talked and listened more to each other, which feels good.'

'Yes, that is good.'

'Yes, and I realized I've misread what I used to call his self-contained style. Tony has been going through his own changes, too. Retirement took him by surprise, I think. I felt that he had become distant – maybe he had – but he wanted to be kind. And now we share our thoughts and our feelings. Isn't that the beginning and end of all of this "getting well" thing?'

'What is?'

'Kindness.'

'Kindness to whom?'

'To myself, for a start.'

'And how would that make you feel?'

'More a winner than a loser, more Laura.'

'That sounds more like it, and it might allow things to come out.'

'Better out than in again, Jim?'

'Yes, the good and the bad.'

'And the ugly! On that topic, myself and Tony are planning a road trip.'

'Where do you want to go?'

'Italy. We're going to see John and the Italian in-laws! Can you imagine? And then we're going to take off by ourselves.'

'To where?'

'Tuscany, Florence, maybe even Venice. Tony's at home right now with his map and highlighter. I don't think he's heard of sat-nav yet!'

'That sounds great, Laura. Are you excited?'

'You know, Jim, I flew thousands of miles for all those years, but I never really went anywhere. Racing at 400 miles an hour but never really moving. I wore a uniform. And someone else set my schedule. Now I'm going to travel to places I want to see. And I'm going to wear what I damn well please.'

Laura's Journey

Laura never anticipated she would have mental health difficulties or an addiction to sedatives or a lifetime of social avoidance. Nevertheless, a disabling pattern of behaviour became entrenched within her life as a result of her experience of a trauma, specifically a rape. This violation became a defining event in her life. All previous attempts at recovery had been fruitless. Until now her attempts at wellness had been incomplete and unsustained. Left without any other effective options, Laura had fallen into the trap of self-medication and she might have remained there had her life not taken an unexpected course.

With ACT, Laura has recovered. She is very well now. Her journey to mental health started with the chance discovery of her access to illegal sources of medication. In legal terms she may not have committed a crime, although those who provided medication on the web may have been criminal. Her discovery led to a crisis, but this opportunity led to her disclosure and her recovery. Laura's assessment led to a detoxification process and ultimately to the modern psychotherapy of Acceptance and Commitment Therapy (ACT). Her individual care plan mapped out a holistic integrated route to wellness and in this partnership was key.

ACT is a modern psychotherapy which, like Behaviour Therapy and Cognitive Behavioural Therapy, places great emphasis on the 'here and now', on the practical and the skills needed to achieve this in the present. It is about living with feelings and emotions rather than disallowing them and it is about being mindful. It involves availability of skilled therapists and an understanding of the value of what ACT calls psychological flexibility:

the ability to reframe our feelings and experiences rather than disown them.

Laura's story illustrates some features of ACT and how it can be mindful and therapeutic. Acceptance of the kind encouraged by ACT is not easy. It means recognizing, acknowledging and owning real distressing feelings and emotions, and then with these feelings taking committed action towards mental health. On the way thoughts and beliefs that previously depressed and disabled Laura were diffused. Through ACT Laura discovered a new meaning for the word 'acceptance' and this gave her painful experience a fresh context. ACT enabled a renewed, more mindful response to her trauma.

The consequence of this acceptance was a different course of action. Genuine acceptance enables action beyond phobic avoidance or chemical numbing of pain. ACT encourages us to 'sit with' suffering rather than to disown it or seek to correct it. By promoting this realism ACT enables a more mindful, kinder reality to emerge. This is the opposite of a denial or a numbed response. With ACT, painful emotions are not 'errors of thinking' as in traditional CBT; they are authentic, integral and genuine parts of experience. The ACT response to this suffering works towards committed action for wellness. Rather than attempt to correct these painful feelings, ACT shows that sometimes it is better to acknowledge them in order to 'unhook' them from our thoughts.

At one stage Laura said she felt as though she were living her life out in a play, as though all of her experience was unreal. This 'de-realization' is a very distressing anxious phenomenon which often goes unrecognized in people with persistent anxiety, particularly after trauma. It may coexist with de-personalization, but together these phenomena represent the sense that the individual and their experience are not real and it is somehow only happening as part of a play or a drama. One does not have to be unwell to experience de-realization/de-personalization. Anyone under extreme stress or exhaustion can experience this, but it is always distressing. Persistent global anxiety such as Laura was describing is a common context for this sensation. The important thing is that Laura was presenting symptoms and challenges which were recognizable and these made sense.

It is not easy to be well when our thoughts and our emotions become fused. ACT teaches that wellness requires fresh thinking. Laura saw only one route to recovery: the removal of her distressing emotions entirely. She saw partial measures as useless. For Laura recovery was all or nothing. Her self-medication offered an illusory route to a distorted idea of wellness. Through ACT Laura learned to accept her feelings and to detach these emotions from her absolute beliefs about recovery and about how things 'had to be'. This diffusion of ideas was helped by consideration of her real values and ambitions. These fresh hopes and dreams had been until now inaccessible. A sense of her own self-worth and the prospect of a more meaningful relationship became possible because of this new reality.

No one defined wellness for Laura. It remains a personal thing and not something easily described, still less prescribed. For me as a doctor, the aim of mental healthcare includes the reduction of suffering, the management of pain and, ideally, the removal of illness, but these medical agendas tend to approach wellness in terms of opposition to pathology rather than the description of a life well lived. The medical model is of value, but it provides a very poor outline of recovery, a bit like a photographer's negative or, at very best, a monochrome picture.

The modern therapeutic team does not attempt to limit the definition of wellness or direct people to one goal. Men and women in therapy drive their own recovery and they identify its goals. My patients encourage me to have a different perspective and so with imagination and kindness this becomes something more than a colourless silhouette. As Jonathan Swift put it, 'Vision is the ability to see the invisible.' Sometimes this wisdom is the ability to visualize what others cannot yet see. At the time of mental distress, this unseen vision is the prospect of wellness. We all need to be reminded of that potential, and so we need to speak up for it wherever we can.

That is one reason why communication helps. ACT provides a

therapeutic conversation not for the amusement of the voyeur. The dialogue of recovery in ACT is more than just the ventilation of distress. These modern therapies show that talking alone is not sufficient to bring about recovery, but communication can create the potential for committed action and that brings wellness with it.

Our role is to provide time and space for such communication in the belief that wellness can re-form. On the journey to recovery, many varied opportunities for engagement may be needed, with many new forms of care. Rarely a period of sanctuary may be necessary – but if this care is to be legitimate it must be based on evidence and determined by human rights.

Ultimately, Laura recovered with the right support, and so when her recovery came, a new vista was apparent to someone who previously saw no hope. The end of her therapy became a new beginning. Wellness through ACT was rediscovered by building upon acceptance and the belief that recovery can follow mental breakdown just as night follows day. Sometimes recovering wellness is less about the advice we give each other and more about the acceptance that we give to ourselves.

Robert and Barbara

ROBERT IS FIFTY-NINE YEARS old. He is a refuse collector and a widower. He was referred to me by his GP, who gave me a very brief outline of his background. Robert had two sons, both of whom were now living in Australia. His only other relative, his younger sister Barbara, with whom he had a close relationship, was very concerned about him.

Robert's wife, Marie, had died ten years earlier as a result of liver cancer arising from hepatitis C. Her death was one of many associated with what in Ireland became known as the 'anti-D – hepatitis C – scandal'. Anger had become an issue for Robert, along with anxiety and depression. The GP noted: 'Robert is severely depressed . . . he has already survived one suicide attempt. Robert is an alcoholic.'

Robert and Barbara's Initial Assessment

The first meeting with someone seeking mental healthcare is always the most important and often the most difficult. It is frequently where unforeseen challenges are highlighted and where the barriers to care are described for the first time. The beginning and ending of therapy is so important because these points in the therapeutic relationship determine the whole course of therapy – whether it will progress or not.

Robert did not want to see me. The reason he came to me was because his sister, Barbara, wanted me to see him and so he felt he had no choice but to go along with her. Barbara was at her wits' end trying to get her brother to stop drinking. She was also finding it challenging to get professional help for him. She had finally prevailed upon her GP to write the referral letter after Robert had made a suicide attempt, but still Robert's engagement with treatment and therapy was not established.

None of this was known to me when Robert and Barbara first arrived. Robert's alcoholism, his bereavement, his suicidal behaviour and his traumatic stress reaction following an accident at work unfolded with his history. The real agenda of our first meeting and of every first meeting was to establish the boundaries of engagement, to begin the building of trust and to offer the hope of a genuine plan for care.

Since the first meeting is a source of apprehension for all those seeking care and a challenge for all those providing it, nothing is achieved when a hostile relationship emerges or when trust is shattered. At our first meeting Robert's demeanour was defensive throughout: his responses were angry and he showed that he felt his situation was hopeless. Barbara described the devastation to her family caused by the death of her sister-in-law Marie and how her brother's grief had led him to a dependence on alcohol.

Addictions can make life very difficult for family, friends and even the community of the abuser, and so the misery of substance abuse is always about more than the primary addicted individual. While resistance to recovery is characteristic for the addicted individual, those close to them often lack the necessary skills to act effectively. The traditional response to this therapeutic challenge has been to advise the community simply to wait for their addicted family member or neighbour to come to their own senses, to allow them to hit 'rock bottom'. Unfortunately this approach left very many people hopelessly to their own fate.

As we have already seen Behaviour Therapy can help an individual to overcome some very distressing psychological problems. It helped Sarah to overcome her fear of contamination, in particular her fear of dog faeces (see Chapter 3, Sarah's Story). This success in one area of her life helped her to regain her independence and rediscover the rest of her life, free of avoidance.

But suppose someone has a more complex behavioural problem. What if a person's psychological difficulty involves more than reflex anxiety leading to avoidance? Can Behaviour Therapy do anything for a problem that involves more than a set of visceral reactions such as palpitations, panic anxiety and avoidance? Such a complex behaviour problem is posed where an addiction or the abuse of a substance is involved. Is it possible for someone to unlearn complex behaviours and instead become conditioned to more healthy ones?

Research suggests that in certain circumstances conditioning of complex behaviours such as addiction is possible. This kind of learning requires a more involved form of Behaviour Therapy technically known as operant conditioning. I prefer to call this therapy 'the conditioning of choices'.

In operant conditioning, the therapist's aim is not simply to *disable* avoidance but instead to *enable* choice of a greater range of behavioural options. Operant conditioning was first described by B. F. Skinner in the 1930s and soon its potential became clear. By selectively rewarding certain behavioural choices, it conditioned them. This conditioning increased the attraction of some choices and diminished the attraction of others. The research showed how association of one choice with a significant reward enlarges its appeal and thus renders the conditioned behaviour more likely to occur.

Some of the techniques of Behaviour Therapy have been harnessed to good effect by one of the most exciting modern post-CBT psychotherapies. It is called CRAFT – or Community Reinforcement Approach and Family Training.

Community Reinforcement Approach and Family Training (CRAFT)

CRAFT is a therapeutic response to a question very frequently asked: How can family members learn to cope with their loved one's continued substance abuse? The frustration felt by family members is often extreme. Traditional therapists emphasize the powerlessness of individuals in this situation, but recent evidence suggests that family and community members are not completely powerless. The truth is we can learn. In certain circumstances the historical advice to 'completely detach and let go' may actually do more harm than good.

Robert Myers, the pioneer of CRAFT therapy, calls these family and community members Concerned Significant Others, or CSOs. In our centre CRAFT is delivered as an eight-week family training programme specifically designed for CSOs living with addiction.[1]

Family members can play a powerful role in reducing their loved one's harmful drinking (or harmful using) and CSOs do this by learning to engage the addicted individual while at the same time improving their own emotional, physical and social wellbeing. CRAFT teaches CSOs practical skills and applies them whether or not their loved one is in treatment or resisting it.

CRAFT therapy has two expressed aims. The first is to improve the mental health and wellbeing of the CSO, and the second is to engage the substance user in an effective therapy. A CRAFT therapist working within a multidisciplinary team supports the CSO. It has always been known that substance abuse and misuse have negative impacts on the user, but we also know that misuse of substances can have an even greater negative impact on the substance abuser's family, friends and community. The scale of familial distress, financial problems and social difficulties caused by alcohol abuse and addiction is underestimated. The same is true of the aggression and interpersonal violence arising from substance misuse. Alcohol abuse is associated with many physical and mental health problems, including depression, post-traumatic stress disorders and anxiety. As family members, colleagues and friends, CSOs typically spend years longing for an end to this abusive disruption in their life and so they also long for

[1] R. J. Meyers, J. E. Smith and D. N. Lash, 'The Community Reinforcement Approach', *Recent Developments in Alcoholism*, 16, 2003, pp. 183–95.

the restoration of their mental and physical health. They too are in search of a life well lived.[2]

According to research, less than 6 per cent of people with alcohol misuse enter into any effective treatment. This refusal to engage persists despite the negative effects that continued alcohol misuse has in so many people's lives. Instead CRAFT proposes that a substance abuser can be conditioned and thus become more likely to enter therapy. Greater engagement in recovery increases the chances of the addicted individual overcoming the abuse of substances.

CRAFT has three main goals:

1. To reduce the loved one's harmful drinking/using
2. To engage the loved one in treatment
3. To improve the physical, emotional and social wellbeing of the CSO

CRAFT empowers the CSO to influence change. It trains the CSO in new behavioural skills and, in doing so, it aims to improve the CSO's quality of life. CRAFT prepares the CSO and the addict for engagement with treatment.

The rationale for the treatment of addiction via therapeutic work with the relative/CSO may be counter-intuitive, but several factors point to the value of this advance. CSOs have unequalled access to the addicted individual and the CSO is often the person in most need of practical help, whether this arises from domestic violence, financial problems or conflict. However, rather than feeling the urgency of these challenges, CSOs experience frustration and disappointment in the face of their loved one's continued substance abuse.

CRAFT seeks to address this by encouraging greater communication within a family still struggling with addiction

---

[2] A popular and engaging description of the therapy can be found in Brenda L. Wolfe and Robert J. Meyers, *Get Your Loved One Sober: Alternatives to Nagging, Pleading, and Threatening*, Hazeldon.

and substance misuse.[3] Together with the CSO, the CRAFT therapist works to develop a detailed treatment package, a specific 'road map' towards recovery. This blueprint is designed to increase the wellbeing of the CSO and thus to condition the substance user to engage with therapy. Tackling the problems of substance misuse in the community using CRAFT means starting with the CSO. It is an effective therapy that identifies a new avenue to the life well lived.

Robert and Barbara's Journey Begins

Tuesday, 20 January 2015

Robert and Barbara arrive together for this meeting. Robert is restless and ill at ease, like a man who could explode at any moment. It is Barbara who speaks first.

'Bob, we are here now. You may as well tell the doctor how you are.'

There is a pause to allow Robert to speak, but he remains silent.

'Doctor, or professor – what am I supposed to call you? I am Barbara, by the way.'

'Doctor will do fine, Barbara. How can I help?'

'Bob's not going to tell you, but I will if you like. You already have his doctor's letter, so you know about his problem.'

'Yes, I have read the referral letter, but I would much rather hear the story from you.'

'The problem is Bob's been drinking so much. He has been through a terrible time over the past few years. It's bad enough that he's lost his wife, but now he's had this accident at work too.'

'Bob, do you want to talk to me about that?'

---

[3] R. J. Meyers, W. R. Miller, J. E. Smith and J. S. Tonigan, 'A randomized trial of two methods for engaging treatment-refusing drug users through concerned significant others', *Journal of Consulting and Clinical Psychology*, Vol. 70(5), Oct. 2002, pp. 1182–5.

'My name's Robert, only Babs gets to call me Bob. Anyway, there is no point in talking. It's no use.'

'Sorry, Robert, but actually it might help to talk about it.'

'Why should I tell you about it anyway? It's just a waste of your time. I'm only here because Babs insisted on it – she's my only sister – but what's done is done. Marie – that's my wife – she's dead. The boys had to go away. And now my work has done this to me.'

'Who has done this to you? What have they done?'

'So you really want the whole story? The whole thing?'

'Yes, I'm here for you, to listen to it all.'

'In an hour – in fifty minutes or whatever it is? Well, I'm not up for it. I'm tired.'

'Hold on now, Bob. The doctor can't help you unless he knows what's happened to you. Maybe I'll tell the story for you – if that's all right with you, doctor?'

'If Robert is OK with it, that might work.'

'Knock yourselves out.'

'Bob works for the council and he was clearing up the Christmas trees, you know, at the depot. I'm right in saying this, Bob? You put your hand into a clump of trees, didn't you? They didn't give you the right gloves, did they? And then something stuck into you.'

'Yes, at first I thought it was the needles of the trees. They hadn't given us the proper gloves. I was always on to them about that. But they said there was never enough in the budget.'

'There's enough in the budget now, isn't there, Bob? They've given the men the right gloves now! Anyway, the long and the short of it is, doctor, he got stabbed with a dirty needle – it must have been a heroin addict's dirty syringe.'

'That must have been awful, Robert. What happened then?'

'What more is there to say? The needle stabbed me, I called to the lads, they brought me to hospital. Then there was all the usual drill: blood tests and investigations. I waited six months before I knew I was fully in the clear.'

'But, Bob, you are in the clear now. They gave you the all-clear months ago.'

'I may be in the clear now, Babs, but I'm destroyed. It has been a bloody nightmare. It was like Marie's death all over, how could this be happening again?'

'Bob, you have had much more than your fair share. I know that.'

'Don't you get it, Babs? My head is wrecked. I haven't been able to sleep for months. I just keep thinking about it over and over in my mind. And you know that's not the worst of it.'

'What's the worst of it, Robert?'

'The worst thing was when I went and took an overdose of tablets. I still feel very guilty. I shouldn't have done that. I just wanted to die, and I couldn't even get that right.'

'Doctor, I found him unconscious – flat out. It's true, he'd taken an overdose. I rang the ambulance in a panic, then I went with him to the hospital. It was a close thing for a while.'

'Robert, what do you remember about the overdose?'

'I only remember some of it. Of course I knew what I was doing. I wasn't even that drunk.'

'And are you safe now, Robert?'

'You mean, am I suicidal? Well, for your information I am "safe" now, as you put it. I'm not suicidal anyway. Sure I wish I was dead, but I'm not going to do anything about it. Now I just drink.'

'I see, Robert, and what does drink do for you? What do you like about drinking?'

'You think I like drinking, do you? No, there's nothing about the drink I like.'

'So why do you drink?'

'I drink to forget. I drink for oblivion.'

'But, Bob, your drinking has to stop. You can't go on like this. It's destroying all our lives!'

'Look, Babs, don't start this fight again. I'm sick of all the rows. I'm not up to it, and I'm not interested.'

'Doctor, you've got to help him.'

'Look, Babs – doctor – it's like this: I'm done here. None of you can help me.'

138

'Ah, Bob, don't go like this.'

'I have to go. I'm not putting up with your guilt trip any longer.'

'Robert, can I talk to Barbara some more? Is that OK with you, if I talk about Barbara's problems and yours? How would you feel about that?'

'At this stage, I don't care. Do what you want. Knock yourself out.'

Robert leaves the room and Barbara sits quietly for some time. She becomes very upset.

'What am I going to do now, doctor? Is there nothing you can do to help Bob?'

'Maybe Robert's just not ready yet.'

'But something has to be done. You have to help him. You can't abandon him. Is there nothing you can do?'

'Maybe there is. It is possible we could start by helping you, Barbara, and that might help Robert. It could take some time, but do you think you would come back to me about this? There are people on my team who would be ready to talk to you about it.'

'I am not sure about this. Talking to *me* isn't what I had in mind at all.'

'Why don't you talk to your GP about it and then we can take it from there?'

Tuesday, 17 February 2015

Barbara returns alone. Although she is concerned that Robert is not involved in these sessions, she is interested to see how effective a therapy like CRAFT could be and wants to know how it might be possible for her to make a positive impact on Robert's recovery by attending treatment herself.

'Good to see you again, Barbara. Thank you for coming.'

'Look, doctor, I got that letter from my GP and I have come back. But as far as I'm concerned it's not *me* that needs your help.

Bob needs someone like you to help him. I can't hold him up by myself, you know?'

'Barbara, why don't we talk a bit more about Robert's drinking?'

'Well, if you want. I suppose . . . I've tried everything else.'

'Why do you think Robert will not come to see me?'

'Alcohol! It's taken him over. He doesn't seem to care any more, you know?'

'It's very hard to reach out to someone who won't accept your help.'

'But that's not good enough, doctor. It's too easy for you to say, "You were offered an appointment and you didn't come."'

'What else can we say, Barbara?'

'That's just it. You don't know, you can't see it because you're too close to all of this. You're part of the system. But there's something wrong with the system. The way I see it Bob can't be left to just sink to the bottom. I've told everyone that his life is in danger. It looks to me like nobody wants to know.'

'And so now you're Robert's only champion?'

'Doctor, I love my brother. I'm not ready to give him up. I'm all he's got, you know?'

'And what about his two boys in Australia? How are they?'

'Since the accident the Skypes are getting fewer. Bob just seems to have lost interest. He used to look forward to the weekly Skype so much. But now . . .'

'Do the boys support him in other ways?'

'Yes, they're good lads, in fairness. But there's nothing here for them. Bob insists on them not wasting their money, "travelling halfway around the world to visit their sad old da", he says. He tells them, "I'm fine, don't worry about me. Go build your new life. Get away from this kip." But they know something's up with him.'

'And do you keep in touch with them, Barbara?'

'Yeah, I still Skype them regularly enough. I love them like they were my own. They lost their mother too. They keep in touch as much as they can. And they are worried. I feel sorry for them. But what can they do from Australia?'

'It can't be easy on them either, Barbara, can it?'

'Well, they're still young men. They will always remember when they lost their mother. It was desperate. Just desperate.'

'Does it really have to be that bad now, Barbara?'

'Of course it does! What do I have to say to you? Do I have to keep telling you that he is suicidal? Is that what it takes to get help for him?'

'Robert's safety is important. And so is yours, Barbara.'

'I don't think so. I don't think anyone would give a toss if he did try to kill himself again – apart from me and the two lads. So it's my job to shield them from all of this and try to hold Bob up. It's a daily battle. My head is wrecked. Why is it so hard to get help for somebody in this day and age?'

'But you're here now, Barbara. That's a start, isn't it?'

'Too many young people are having to leave to make a living. And the ones in charge here are just covering their own arses, you know? Maybe Bob is right, maybe it is a kip.'

'We've all felt like that, Barbara. It's OK to be angry, frustrated. That's all perfectly real.'

'I'll tell you what's real: my brother needs help. He looked after me when we were growing up. And I'm not going to fail him when he needs me most. I'll move heaven and earth if I have to!'

'Barbara, maybe there are things we can do for you. Can I talk to you about a new therapy we have called CRAFT?'

'But you're not hearing me, doctor. *I* don't need the therapy, *Bob* does.'

'But with CRAFT, Barbara, we might be able to help him *through* you. Will you let me try and explain? Maybe if we could rediscover your role in Robert's life, we could help both of you to have better lives. After all, you've done so much for each other already.'

'Maybe so.'

'I bet you're fed up pleading with him and fighting?'

'Oh, for sure. I'm so tired of that. Talk about beating your head off a brick wall.'

'And you want your brother to have a better life?'

'Of course – that's why I'm here.'

'So things have to change, don't they? The pleading is not working. The good thing is that there are alternatives.'

'What are they? I've done the Al-Anon. Don't get me wrong, they have been brilliant, they saved my life. But there's one thing they tell me to do and I won't do it. They say I have to "learn how to detach, with love". But I won't do that. Bob's the only family I have.'

'Maybe we could start Robert's recovery in a different way, by changing your life?'

'And how would that help Bob?'

'Imagine if you could reclaim your good life. Instead of arguing and pleading with him, you might be happier. In some way Robert could choose to be part of that better life, couldn't he?'

'Are you saying it's my fault?'

'No, not at all. It's nobody's fault. But supposing you and Robert could both have better lives, what would that look like for you and for him?'

'My happiness is his. I can't be happy if I just sit back, detach and lose him altogether.'

'But maybe your happiness could help him, too. Maybe that's where we could make a difference. Would you like to think about your wellbeing?'

'I really don't understand any of this. It's not making much sense to me. It's just such a pity that he isn't here. You will see him some day, won't you?'

'I will see him, of course, when he chooses to come. But there's so much you and I can achieve in the meantime while we're here waiting for Robert to make that choice. Maybe you could come and talk to me about Robert. I'd like to know what kind of man he really is. And we could work together so that we have an understanding of Robert and of his drinking. Together we could draw a road map to his recovery and yours. Barbara, if you come back to me, we can talk some more about this plan we call CRAFT.'

'What choice do I have? I have to do something. For Robert.'

Thursday, 5 March 2015

Barbara remains apprehensive about attending therapy. She finds it hard to prioritize her own happiness.

'Why don't you tell me, what kind of a man is your brother? Talk to me about Robert in your own words.'

'In my own words?'

'Yes, in your own words. Take your time. I'd like to know more about you and your brother.'

'OK, doctor. It seems a little weird to be asking me about him, but if you think it'll help.'

'It could be very helpful, Barbara.'

'Marie – that's Bob's wife – she died ten years ago this December. From liver cancer, you know? Three weeks before Christmas, to be exact. Leaving Bob with two thirteen-year-old boys. How cruel was that?'

'Yes, that must have been devastating.'

'God, we were in such shock at first. Rushing around trying to organize a funeral. And shielding the boys from the truth of it.'

'And how did you manage, Barbara?'

'I don't know. Your guess is as good as mine. I remember stopping and staring at the Christmas lights in town. I just broke down in tears, there in the street. People were looking at me, holding their shopping bags. So I just said to myself: *Keep going. Bob and the boys need you now. You have to step up.*'

'And that's what you did, isn't it? You stepped up.'

'What else could I do? Anyway, Christmas was a bit of a blur that year. Lots of people, neighbours and family, around the house. "Sorry for your loss" and all that. Bob was like a zombie. The boys just went very quiet. Confused, numb-like, you know?'

'Sometimes, Barbara, we'd all like to cancel Christmas. Maybe we should . . .'

'Well, I suppose there's no good time for something like that to happen, doctor. Anyway, a few weeks passed and we were heading into the spring. Not so many of the neighbours around at this stage. The wake was well over. People move on to the next thing, naturally enough.'

'And was Robert's drinking obvious at that time, Barbara?'

'No, not really. Not yet. Just the normal drinking. He was angry, though. We all were. Marie was such a young woman. And now she was gone. A good wife and mother gone before her time. And she did nothing wrong, nothing to deserve this. You're meant to be able to trust these hospitals . . . Anyway, Bob was fuming for ages. Then he just seemed to get lonely, like.'

'Lonely?'

'Yeah, quieter. Not as angry. He stopped talking about the scandal.'

'And it was a scandal, wasn't it?'[4]

'An absolute disgrace! The government should be ashamed of itself – all those people getting hepatitis C from infected blood. Marie got it from a transfusion after the boys were born. Imagine that? You're supposed to be able to *trust* these hospitals. It's just disgusting what they did. And we were not the only family that lost everything.'

'It must have been very distressing, Barbara.'

'It was. And do you know how many people died of liver cancer as a result? I read it in the paper the other day: 260 people.[5] What sort of a place is this, doctor? Nobody was held responsible for Marie's death. They all kept their jobs and their pensions. Don't get me wrong, we got some compensation. But we never got a sincere apology, and in any case an apology wouldn't bring Marie back. What use is thirty pieces of silver anyway?'

'Was the compensation any good to Marie?'

'She did put it to good use. She used it to raise the boys. And she used it to help out everyone close to her: Bob and the

[4] The 'anti-D – hepatitis C – scandal' arose when many Irish women were given contaminated blood products post-partum by the Irish Blood Transfusion Service. As the scandal unfolded the real cost for the mothers emerged. See 'Anti-D scandal was a bloody disgrace' by Caroline O'Doherty, *Irish Examiner*, 21 February 2014.

[5] 'At least 260 deaths in 20 years since hepatitis C scandal erupted. Report reveals health consequences of contaminated blood products supplied by State.' *The Irish Times*, 30 July 2015.

boys and me. That's how I'm here. I couldn't afford this otherwise.'

'It's good you're here, Barbara. So, you were talking to me about Robert's drinking.'

'Yeah, the heavy drinking started then – after the anger.'

'And could you recognize it when Robert had been drinking heavily?'

'Sometimes. But what difference does that make?'

'Well, it might help us to look at things you've tried to change and see what worked, what was less successful.'

'You mean like the old serenity prayer? "God grant me the serenity to accept the things I cannot change, the courage . . ." and all of that?'

'Maybe, Barbara.'

'Sorry, but I'm all out of serenity, doctor. I'll tell you that for nothing.'

'That's understandable, Barbara. But maybe you can describe for me what happens on a typical drinking day for Robert?'

'I challenge him. He denies it. I give him the benefit of the doubt. But he still drinks. The same pattern, again and again. But every time he's drunk something bad happens. I'm kind of left there, hoping that he'll hit his rock bottom, you know?'

'And when you argue what happens?'

'Ah, it's always the same. I'll push him too much and that's his trigger to march straight back to the pub or to his flat and hit the bottle again.'

'Maybe, Barbara, we can change things for you and then see how everything else changes?'

'Chance would be a fine thing! But one thing's for sure: I can't go on like this too much longer, doctor.'

'Let's do something a little different. Here's a blank sheet of paper and a pen. Can you try and write out the last argument you had with Robert?'

'Write it?'

'Yes, it might be worthwhile. What did he say, how did you react?'

'I can tell you much quicker than I can write it.'

'That might be true, but this way we can both have a real look at it and then we can maybe write a new script – with different words, softer language, some alternatives?'

'Well, maybe. Our old rows are going nowhere, I know that.'

'You know your brother better than anyone alive. Couldn't we use that knowledge to give us some new tools and some new hope?'

'If you're talking about some kind of therapy, I need the nuts and bolts. You can talk to other people about hope and making big changes, but it just doesn't seem real to me, where I am. I don't need false promises.'

'There's nothing false about this. I am going to ask you to see Imelda. She's my colleague here and she's a CRAFT therapist. I would like you to talk to her. With Imelda's help and mine, you're going to feel better yourself. That could make a big difference for Robert, too.'

'But how will I be helping Bob?'

'Well, first of all we will help you. That would be worthwhile, wouldn't it? And that might give Robert some alternatives. It will certainly give you some options. The hope is for a better life – for you and Robert.'

'My happiness is way down the list of my priorities, doctor. But a better life for both of us does sound good, especially if you say it'll help Bob.'

Thursday, 19 March 2015

Barbara has started attending CRAFT sessions, but her focus remains on Robert and his interests rather than hers.

'Doctor, you know you mentioned this list of things that I think trigger Bob's drinking?'

'Yes, Barbara. Have you been working on it?'

'Well, I took your advice and joined the CRAFT group. I had a long chat with Imelda and she helped me to write up the list.'

'That's good.'

'You can see it is not that long. "Anger" and "grief" are on the top. My "encouragement" is there, too. That one seems to drive him mad altogether. Quiet mad, you know? He'll just walk off. He's a gentle giant, he really is.'

'I see you have the words "just move on" on your list, Barbara. Can you explain that to me?'

'Well, he hates anyone saying he should "just move on".'

'He's right, though, isn't he? People can't just move on. After all, he has lost his wife.'

'Not just lost, she was taken from us. He feels she was taken from him. Did I tell you he tried to overdose too?'

'Yes, Barbara. We need to talk a bit more about that. When did it happen?'

'After the accident at work.'

'Robert spoke about the accident when you both came to see me.'

'Well, you know he works for the council. I think he must be nearly twenty-five years working for the city. He got the job after he came back from London. He was on the buildings for years, since he was sixteen.'

'Sounds like Robert worked hard, Barbara?'

'That's for sure. It's been hard-going, rain or shine, but he never complained. Got on great with the lads. The other lads would kind of look up to him, you know? He's a lot more than just a bin man, as some people might call him.'

'Absolutely. They respected him, Barbara?'

'That's right. And before all this he respected himself.'

'So where did you and Robert grow up?'

'We grew up together in Dublin, the inner city, in the flats. True Blues, Up the Dubs, you know? He's nearly ten years older than me. A great big brother, you know, always looking out for me.'

'It's good to have a guardian like that growing up, isn't it?'

'He was a good footballer, too, but he didn't stick at it. He always loved running, though. Always kept that going. Always very fit – until the last few years.'

'Was he a bit of a sportsman?'

'Oh yeah. I was devastated when he went to England for work. I was only six, but I remember the loss I felt. Devastated. But he had to go. I thought I'd never see him again. But he'd come back for Christmases and weddings and funerals. And when he got the job with the council here full-time I think I was happier than anyone else in the whole world.'

'Did Robert get an education?'

'No, back then there was no money for that, he had to leave school early and get a job. But he's clever, one of the smartest guys I know. Self-taught, you know? Have you ever seen the lads down the Phoenix Park on a Sunday morning, flying the model planes?'

'Yes, many times.'

'Well, you would've seen Bob then. He used to be the main man down there. He's just brilliant at building those planes. They say he could make anything fly.'

'Sounds like a great pastime, Barbara. Did you ever fly the planes?'

'God, no. I'd have probably crashed into the obelisk thing – or killed a deer or something! I'd often go down to watch Bob and the two boys there, though.'

'A lovely way to spend a Sunday morning.'

'Yeah, they're some of the happiest times I can remember.'

'Barbara, what kind of a person is Robert?'

'You've asked me that question before. I've thought a lot about it. I would say he's very kind, a very intelligent person. A gentle giant, like I said. He's street smart, too. You don't have to have a formal education to be smart. There is a difference, you know?'

'Absolutely, Barbara, of course.'

'And he really cared for Marie. Loved her. Bob says they killed her when they gave her the infected blood after the twins were born. And then they tried to cover it up. I say they might not have intended to, but they infected her all the same. It was bad blood. They should have known.'

'But the two boys, they came through OK?'

'Yeah, I suppose so. They were grand, like, thank God. Marie was devoted to them. And still she had the hep C hanging over her all the time. She was tired a lot but a great mother to those boys. Spirits always high, no matter what. She was always campaigning for survivors of hep C. She ran the marathon with Bob I don't know how many times. Raised tens of thousands for cancer, I'd say, you know?'

'Is that how he kept his spirits up?'

'For sure. Bob always kept himself busy. If he wasn't training for a marathon, he was in his workshop fixing up a plane for the weekend.'

'And then, when Marie died?'

'Things just fell apart. Bob felt – still feels – Marie was taken away from him by criminals and yet nobody was held responsible. Nothing has been learned.'

'We're all trying to learn, but it's hard to change the health system, isn't it?'

'I expected you'd be defending the system.'

'No, Barbara, not at all. I don't mean to defend any system.'

'Well, who cares now. I have no time for systems. They're not alive. They don't get sick or depressed or die. But people do.'

'Do you think Robert would like an apology, even if it was from the system?'

'What value is an apology now – to Bob, or Marie, or even me?'

'You're very angry about all of this, Barbara, aren't you?'

'You're damn right I'm angry. And you would be too, if you were on the receiving end of any of this.'

'That's true.'

'Bob is alone. Except for me . . .'

'Barbara, will you talk to me some more about Robert's accident at work?'

'Like he told you himself a few weeks ago, he was doing a bit of tidying up around the depot and he went to pick up a bunch of Christmas tree branches, to put through the shredder, you know? Then he got this jab on his right hand, through his glove.'

'His hands were pierced?'

'That's right. And when he saw the dirty syringe needle sticking out of his fingers, he says his heart just dropped. I told you about the gloves, didn't I? They have them all wearing those fancy new gloves now. Covering their arses as usual.'

'And Robert went for all the blood tests?'

'Yeah, HIV, hep C, the whole lot.'

'And the results came back OK?'

'It took weeks, but he finally got the all-clear. Nobody could reassure him, though. He was terrified. He thought what had happened to Marie was happening to him.'

'History repeating itself?'

'That's what he thought. He was convinced he had hep C or HIV. He used to say that he could feel his blood all poisoned.'

'And how did he cope?'

'He took a big step down. More drinking, worse depression, and then in the end he took the overdose. I feel so guilty about that overdose.'

'Why should you feel guilty about Robert's overdose? You were the one trying to help him, weren't you?'

'But they were my pills. I didn't tell you, did I? He did it by taking my pills.'

Tuesday, 14 April 2015

Barbara describes her own experience of depression and agrees that CRAFT therapy is helping her to be more positive. She sees no improvement in her brother's condition, though, and remains anxious about him.

'I didn't really want to get into all of this, but Imelda, your CRAFT person, says I've got to. So yes, I have been depressed. I've been on antidepressants for a long time. Well, I suppose since shortly after my mother died.'

'I'm sorry to hear of your mother's death. When was that, Barbara?'

'A couple of years before Marie passed – 2003.'

'Were you close with your mother?'

'Yeah, well, I suppose; we weren't like sisters, as some women would say about their mothers. She was in her forties when I came along – a surprise baby, you might call me. Bob used to say I was a Christmas sherry baby. That used to make me laugh.'

'So you were unexpected?'

'Yeah, not in the plan. But I was a happy baby. Bob raised me really. Unusual for a boy, I know, but he was very responsible for a young lad. My parents worked all the time, we'd only see them in the evenings. We sort of brought each other up.'

'So your mother must have died quite young, Barbara?'

'Yeah, both of my parents died young really – and suddenly, you know? I never had to care for them in their old age because they didn't make it that far.'

'It must have been difficult for you, losing your parents like that?'

'Ah, it was, yeah. I loved Ma and Da. But times were very different then. There was always a distance between me and Ma. Not like a coldness, don't get me wrong, just a distance, you know?'

'Raising a family – "parenting", as they say – it was different in those days, don't you think?'

'Yeah, my parents didn't expect anything much from life either. They just worked all the time, or so it seemed to me, and when they'd get home they'd be wrecked. Me and Bob kind of just got on with it, without them. Ma was quiet – they never seemed to talk to each other much – and Da was fond of his pint. Ma rarely drank, just the odd sherry. Like I said, at Christmas!'

'Was your father's drinking a problem back then, Barbara?'

'No, I wouldn't say that, doctor. He was no different than all the other men around. It was what men did, I suppose.'

'I see.'

'Anyway, I got a good chance at education – a better chance than Bob got, that's for sure. I had a couple of good teachers. I was smart, you know? I remember one teacher in particular, Miss Martin. She was younger than most of the others and she used to say to me, "You can be anything you want to be – anything!" I loved that, I just loved to hear that. It gave me real confidence, you know?'

'It's amazing how much difference a good teacher can make to our childhood, isn't it?'

'Yeah, she really helped me. College was never going to happen – one step at a time and all that. But I did land a good job in Clerys department store in town, in the children's department. I've always loved my job, dressing the kids for communions and things like that. I love the kids. Mind you, they're getting bolder these days. But I love to see their little faces delighted with their new outfits.'

'And so do you have any idea why it was that you got depressed?'

'I'm not into self-analysis, doctor, and I don't have the time or the money to be obsessed about my mental health. I'm not like some of these celebs. Do you ever notice they never seem to be depressed for the photo shoots?'

'Forgive me, Barbara. I never meant to suggest that this was self-indulgent. I'm just curious to know how your depression might have come about, you know?'

'Look, doctor, I can't explain it. I don't have a big secret from my childhood or anything like that. I got a good start, a chance at education. I see my life as being lucky, you know? Lucky enough anyways. Could have been a lot worse, I know that.'

'And do you remember a time when you didn't feel depressed?'

'I don't know, it just kind of . . . It came on me, you know? A bit like being fifty or something. I'm fifty next year. One day you wake up and you're fifty! Like, how did that happen? That's what the depression was like for me too, if that makes sense.'

'Talk to me some more about your depression. Can you describe it?'

'Well, you wake up and think, *I feel so sad*. How did that happen? Why does it happen to anyone?'

'There is no one single reason to be depressed. Sometimes it's about lots of things coming together.'

'Sometimes I think it all started when Bob went to England for work. I felt that I had to grow up overnight. It was really hard on me.'

'Is there anyone else in your family with depression?'

'Yes, of course there is. I mean, what about my Bob? Have you forgotten why I'm here?'

'Of course not, sorry. I was wondering whether in your family there was a general tendency to depression?'

'Because depression runs in families?'

'Yes, it can do. But that doesn't explain it entirely.'

'And so if it's not in my genes, then you think my childhood might explain it?'

'Yes, that too, to some degree. After all, you lost your guardian, Barbara? That is what he was, wasn't he?'

'Yes, I was still a baby. Bob wasn't going to be there for me any more. I thought I'd never see him again, and I know he didn't want to go either. He had to, for the work, but he would have preferred to stay.'

'It must have been very hard on you. You were still a child, Barbara. Is that it?'

'Yeah, but what can you do? I just worked hard at school, then I got my job and I guess before I knew it I was all grown up. And then Bob was back.'

'And you were very happy to have Robert back home.'

'God, yeah! Like everyone, I was delighted. But then time seemed to pass so quickly. Bob got married to Marie, the twins were born, then Da died, then Ma died, and then Marie died. And during all that time I must have been getting a little lower each year, a bit like going down stairs, you know?'

'Yes, that feeling must be dreadful. Were there other good people in your life during all that time?'

'Ah, I've always had friends. And I had a few boyfriends. Maybe I should have held on to one or two of them. One in particular – Bob used to say he was a decent lad.'

'And what happened to that relationship, Barbara?'

'Ah, he had to leave, you know, for work as well. He wanted me to go with him. He really did. But I could never leave, not me.'

'Where was he going?'

'Canada. Too far away for me. And besides, I had my parents. I thought I'd have to look after them in their old age. And Marie had just had the twins. I couldn't go.'

'Did you ever see him again, Barbara? What happened?'

'No, he never came back. Not that I know of anyway. Just disappeared. I do think about him from time to time, though. I sometimes imagine what my life would have been like in Canada. But I guess that's stupid talk. You play the hand you're dealt, right?'

'You made some choices.'

'Yes, I did. I suppose I wanted to make my life in Ireland. Bloom where you're planted, my da always said. It isn't just about finding the right man who'll sweep you off your feet. This is my home. I know Bob says this place is a kip, but I've never felt like that. I have no time for politics, but I think you can have a good life here. Staying here was certainly my choice and I don't regret it.'

'In any case, none of that explains why you became depressed, does it, Barbara?'

'No, I've never been able to find a good explanation. For me, depression isn't like that.'

'Talk to me some more about what depression is like for you. Will you tell me?'

'I'd usually be OK during the day, at work and all, but I'd get lonely at night. I've cried myself to sleep more times than, well, I don't know what – sometimes for weeks and nights in a row. But I didn't know why I was so upset. I'd sit up in the bed and shout at myself, *What the hell is wrong with you?!* But when you're depressed the sadness is just so overwhelming, you know, completely eats you up.'

'And how are you today, Barbara?'

'Well, all I can say is that I'm not depressed now.'

'Why is that?'

'Imelda says it's a combination of things and I suppose she is right. I am minding myself. I've done my mindfulness stress-reduction course. I take my meds, of course, and I eat well. I don't drink too much. And I've lots of good friends. I'm in a choir. I keep in touch with people. I'm not some *sad old woman*, you know? I am learning how to stay well, too. I take things one day at a time.'

'So have things improved since you started seeing Imelda and the group?'

'Yes, I have to admit that. Imelda and her CRAFT group have helped me to stop the arguing and the pleading with Bob. She says we can find better alternatives. We do a lot of mindfulness meditation together. I used to read about that but with the group it's really become something that has helped me. I haven't seen any of this helping Bob yet, though. Not really. I'm not sure where it is all going. It shouldn't really be all about me, it's about Bob. I need Bob to get well.'

'I understand that you love your brother. The question is, how are we going to help him to get well? I don't want you to be more frustrated than you have been. All the energy you've put into minding yourself and getting well, all of that is good and it could be helpful for Robert too – if we could just go a little further with it and give him a choice to join you in your wellness.'

'But suppose he doesn't want to join me?'

'But suppose he makes that choice?'

Thursday, 30 April 2015

We talk about the concept of a 'road map', connecting Barbara's recovery to Robert's. We look at the mindful approach offered by CRAFT.

'Bob copes by drinking – it's what he chooses to do. He says he doesn't need any help. He still says the drink helps him. I think it anaesthetizes him. He drinks in the evening and in the morning, in company and alone.'

'And can you always tell when Robert's been drinking?'

'Yeah, Imelda asked me about this. I can tell because his voice changes. And he gets more irritable, you know? He starts giving out more, gets teary and maudlin talking about Marie and about his accident.'

'So you can recognize his drinking signs? That's going to be very helpful.'

'Yes, I am learning they're the times it usually ends in a row. Imelda is telling me that the rows have to stop before it gets out of hand. Still, sometimes I worry that you people think this whole thing is my fault, you know?'

'But it's not your fault, Barbara. We all know this isn't about blaming you.'

'I suppose. Imelda is helping me feel better about that now. I'm not blaming myself as much as I used to. And I have taken her advice to stop pleading with him. However much I want to argue, those days are over.'

'That's got to be good, at least for you. Tell me, Barbara, has Robert ever been violent?'

'No, never. Imelda asked me that too, but there's no danger of that.'

'It is very important to us that you're safe. That's paramount.'

'Well, I am. Bob would never do anything like that to me, drunk or sober. And I would never put up with that.'

'Has Robert ever had any other alcohol-related problems – road traffic accidents, falls, head injuries or fits? Anything like that?'

'No, not unless you count being depressed or not being able to turn up for work. Do you count those things?'

'Yes, we do.'

'And trying to kill himself . . . Do you count that, doctor?'

'Absolutely, of course we do, Barbara.'

'Ah, maybe you think I'm being too hard on you. Making a point! I can see you're not heartless. But, really, what is the use of all of these detailed questions to me about Bob? Granted, I am much better in myself. But what can you do for Bob?'

'Barbara, do you remember we had this conversation last time we met? It's like this. You being well is a first step. Gathering all of the information about Robert's drinking will help you make the next step.'

'And what is the next step?'

'Let's call it the "road map". And with this map, we'll have a way of planning for tomorrow, for your tomorrow and for Robert's as well.'

'Most people say to me I'm wasting my time, no good will happen until Bob hits rock bottom, whenever that happens.'

'The rock bottom approach seems very brutal and very simplistic to me, Barbara. Let's not take that route. Let's take the CRAFT approach, which is very different.'

'So what does CRAFT say is the next step?'

'CRAFT involves you changing your behaviour, Barbara.'

'Jesus, you're not going to tell me now that I'm *enabling* him!'

'No, I'm not saying that, Barbara. Sorry, I don't mean to upset you. Look at it this way, Barbara. Things are better between you and him. Since you've been seeing Imelda at the CRAFT group, you've changed your reactions to him and the rows have stopped. And now you're feeling better.'

'But do you understand, this isn't just an academic exercise for me, you know? I'm here for my brother.'

'Absolutely. I know you are.'

'Can you just promise me one thing, doctor? Will you help him? Will you see him?'

'Of course, if he will see me. After all, he is a free man.'

'Free to kill himself, you mean.'

'Hopefully not. What we are doing is giving him a choice of a better life. And that choice of a better life might include you.'

'I have to get some help for him because he's not going to help himself. He's still drinking. I can't just watch him die. I'm still holding on for him, doctor. Holding on like a loose button. But will holding on be good enough?'

'We have to hope it will be.'

'I just don't know if I'm able to be that hopeful.'

Tuesday, 12 May 2015

Barbara arrives for this session feeling positive. There is a change in her attitude to her wellbeing. She is beginning to see how her positivity can influence the choices Robert is making.

'I used to be very fit, you know? Bob ran the marathons and I used to train with him, many an early morning up in the Phoenix Park with the deer and the mist and all of that. I just love being back running. Feels great.'

'And you're sticking with it, Barbara?'

'Absolutely. Love it. Never feel bad after a run, you know? And all you need is a decent pair of runners.'

'So you're going back to something you love?'

'Definitely. I've been putting my life back together, finding my priorities, doing things I enjoy – not just following some list for wellness advice. I suppose Imelda has helped me change the way I feel about Bob.'

'Yes, Barbara, do you remember when you said your own happiness was down your list of priorities?'

'Sure I do. Funny how that's all changed.'

'And so, is Robert still your priority?'

'Yes, of course he is. It doesn't have to be either/or, does it, doctor?'

'Absolutely not, but you have rediscovered how important it is to feel good yourself.'

'Exactly, doctor. I'd say that.'

'But you still want to help Robert, of course?'

'Yeah, now more than ever. I have been going to the CRAFT group and I'm starting to understand that letting myself go was no good for anyone.'

'And are the other good things that you're doing helping you?'

'Well, the running is for one thing. I like it because it's something Bob and me could do together. It's not just about finding ways to reduce my stress. It'd be great if he would join me.'

'So you're telling me he's probably not going to join your choir, then?'

'No, I can't see that ever happening! He's not the musical type. But he might run with me.'

'And have you asked him to join you for a run?'

'When Imelda suggested that a few weeks back, I thought to myself, *Good luck with that!* But I said I'd chance it anyway.'

'And?'

'At first I got blanked completely. But I didn't let that stop me. Or disappoint me.'

'So you persisted?'

'Yeah, like she said, in a *non-confrontational* way. And lo and behold, I started to get a No, which is better than a blank! And then last week he said to me: "I'll need new runners. I can't find the old ones."'

'Looks like you might be on to something, Barbara.'

'Do you think?'

'He might join you.'

'I hope so.'

Thursday, 28 May 2015

When Barbara returns, she brings Robert with her. She is cheerful and keen to reintroduce him to me. Robert is standing tall now. His face is clean-shaven and his dark hair is brushed well off his face. He greets me warmly before he sits down.

'Robert, you're very welcome back. It is so good to see you again.'

'Hello, doctor. It's good – or I mean, well, I suppose it is good to see you again too.'

'He's here off his own bat too, doctor. I didn't have to drag him here. He suggested it himself, that's the truth.'

'That's great, Barbara. Is there anything in particular you'd like to talk about today, Robert, now that the three of us are here again?'

'Well, that's just it, doctor. There is. You see, it's very strange but something happened. About two weeks ago, was it, Babs?'

'Yeah, Bob, two weeks ago.'

'It's been a dreadful experience, you could say. A horrible one. But it has made things clearer to me, I think.'

'Will you talk about it here, Robert? Would you like to do that?'

'He wants me to be here, doctor. But he wants to tell you himself, about what happened.'

'That's good, Barbara. It's good that we all want to be here.'

'Bob's been doing great recently, doctor. He's been going back to AA and he's even talking about seeing a therapist – maybe somebody like Imelda. That's right, isn't it, Bob?'

'Yeah, that's true, Babs. Things are a bit better. I'm working on it anyway. Look, doctor, I've always known I have an addictive personality: the running, the planes, and then – unfortunately – the drink. So I went back to my AA meetings, you know, to try and get some balance back.'

'That's a fantastic achievement, Robert. You must be very proud.'

'Not proud. Definitely not proud, doctor. I'm taking nothing for granted, but I'm not as sad or as drunk as I was before . . . I'm sorry, doctor. There is something else. I'm not very good at this. Not much of a talker. I hate talking at the meetings too.'

'Don't worry, Bob. I told you the doctor is a good listener. Give him a shot. He might understand.'

'All right, well, the first thing is that I want to apologize for that walkout I did the last time I was here. I want to apologize to you and to Babs. I know she's only trying to help me. But I just get so angry sometimes. I could feel the anger rising in me that day.'

'That's OK, and we don't all have to be talkers, Robert.'

'I wanted to try and explain things to you, doctor. But it's hard for me, you know?'

'I do know that, Robert, and I'm happy to hear whatever it is you want to tell me.'

'When Marie, my wife, was still with us, I used to try and keep fit for the both of us. I used to run marathons, you know, to raise money for liver cancer.'

'I was telling the doctor that before, Bob. You've raised tens of thousands, I'd say.'

'Yeah, anyway, when Marie died it just . . . knocked the stuffing out of me. I felt my heart just burst – like a tyre.'

'It's been dreadful for you, Robert. I know that. But now you're getting back to a healthier life?'

'Yeah, as I said I'm back at the AA meetings. Twice a day there for a while. It was full-on. It's good, though. They help a lot. I know that every day I don't drink is a bonus. I'm feeling a lot better. Apart from the speaking at the meetings. I hate that bit, but I know being there is important.'

'Yes, really great, Robert.'

'Yeah, but that's not what I wanted to tell you. I want to tell you about another thing, something terrible that happened, and it's sort of changed me. I would never have imagined it. It's hard to explain but it made me realize, you know?'

'What is it, Robert?'

'Well, it's something that happened when I started running in our local park again, you know, with Babs, like we used to years ago? Now we go early, before work, so it's still a bit dark or only getting bright. It's the best time of the day. So, the other morning we were just five minutes in when I spotted him. I wasn't 100 per cent sure at first, but it became clear pretty quickly.'

'Who did you spot, Robert?'

'I could see a man. Hanging. He was a young man, I could tell straight away. He was hanging from a tree. Just hanging there. Still. Lifeless.'

'That was an awful discovery to make. Did you see him too, Barbara?'

'I don't wear my glasses when we're out running, doctor. I'm half-blind ordinarily, so I couldn't make it out. But I knew something was up. Bob just stopped dead. "What is it, Bob?" I said. And he said, "Get back – keep away!" And he said, "Call an ambulance. Tell them to come as fast as they can." So I went off to call for help.'

'It was a terrible sight, doctor. I didn't want Babs to see him.'

'So what did you do, Robert?'

'At first I kind of panicked, you know? Next thing I knew I was trying to hold him up, but I couldn't. God, he was stone cold and felt twice the weight he looked. I tried to cut him down then, but I just couldn't. I didn't have anything on me, you know, like a pen-knife or anything. Then I just kind of froze. My feet were rooted to the ground. At that stage it was just me and him. His eyes were open wide. It was awful. And I couldn't do anything for him.'

'And did help arrive, Robert?'

'Yeah, eventually. Felt like an age to me. I could see the ambulance outside the park, flashing lights and all. But they couldn't get through the smaller gates, so they had to turn and go the long way round and in the main entrance. I was left with him for another while – not able to help him. I knew he was long gone already. Eventually they got to us. I stayed through the whole thing, like an eejit, trying to help. But sure, what could be done at that stage?'

'Doctor, I stood well back, you know, until the ambulance lads were done. Then I brought Bob back to my place for a cup of tea. He was desperate upset.'

'It can't have been easy for you either, Barbara.'

'No, but it's over now, the whole thing. No point in getting upset now, Bob. It's finished.'

'I'm not upset, Babs. That's just it. Not any more anyway. That's what I want to tell you both. That's what's so strange about it all. I feel, like, relieved or something. It's very strange, you know?'

'Relieved, Robert?'

'The thing is, right, you both have to understand this. The way I see it, that young man hanging from the tree, he could have been *me*. I could have been him, hanging there, in the dawn, dead. Do you understand?'

'Go on, Robert . . .'

'I tried to kill myself once, doctor, you know? Before, with her pills. I know how it feels to be there. And looking at that young man hanging there, cold, I thought to myself: maybe he is better off.'

'But, Robert, we don't know that?'

'That's the point, I suppose, doctor. You see, I feel like I've died a few times already. And this dead man made me really feel something about it. Looking at the poor fella made me think of Marie. And I thought about Marie and how I know she is also dead . . . I know I must sound terrible.'

'No, Robert, not at all.'

'And I was thinking, like, how – well, you see, I'm not dead. I'm still alive. I'm living. And because I'm living, anything is possible, anything can happen for us.'

'I think I understand, Bob. You're saying we're still together and that's what counts.'

'And we can go on, that's what I mean. And maybe make it better.'

Robert and Barbara's Journey

Recovery really happens. Robert and Barbara have rediscovered a better life, a life well lived, but the question is this: how does recovery happen? The answer to this question is not as straightforward as it might seem.

Let's start with Barbara's story. Hopefully we can agree that Barbara has found a better life. First, Barbara has come to recognize the benefit of being well and this time for herself. Her recovery from depression has not been easy. For Barbara, it involved the difficult task of acknowledging her own needs. Having her own CRAFT therapist made a difference because it allowed her the time and space to focus primarily on these needs. Barbara had experienced much bereavement in her life. Her early childhood separation from Robert was a great loss. As an adult, she lost her parents and her sister-in-law in quick succession. Mourning is one of the deepest paths to melancholia. Barbara dismissed any suggestion that her life would have been happier had she married and emigrated to North America. This was Barbara's choice and she remains adamant it was the right one. She may be right. It is not for us to judge. In any case as a psychiatrist it is not for me to comment. I learned a long time ago that a romantic idea of marriage is no cure for depression. Indeed, it may add to it.

So, with the help of Imelda and her CRAFT group, Barbara rediscovered her well-lived life, living in the present, living mindfully. Now she feels less hesitant about taking time to care for herself. She enjoys her choir, her friends and her exercise. She also finds joy in her work. Of course the future is never certain, but objectively Barbara has gained a great deal. And crucially she renewed and rebalanced her relationship with her brother, Robert.

So, what about Robert? How has CRAFT helped him? Perhaps

vicariously? As he put it, 'I know now that every day that I don't drink is a bonus.' And so it seems this bonus was possible because of the CRAFT approach. Barbara's recovery helped Barbara help Robert and so together (and independently) they discovered a new vision of their future.

CRAFT therapy is another hopeful successor to Behaviour Therapy and Cognitive Behavioural Therapy. CRAFT uses many of the same behavioural techniques, leading to clear planning and preparation of behavioural pathways, the so-called road map. CRAFT also works in a group setting, which increases fellowship and helps maintain motivation. Its use of vicarious learning, the observation by Robert of Barbara's progress, is also a powerful form of conditioning. This provided Robert with an opportunity to make a choice which pleading and nagging had hitherto obscured.

But Robert and Barbara's story also reveals the limitations of an exclusively behavioural understanding of mental recovery in human beings. We are none of us creatures in a box responding simply to reward or punishment. We are not ordinary mammals open to straightforward manipulation. Unlike other creatures, we think as well as feel – and uniquely we can identify with others. This identification mobilizes us to empathize and so to move beyond our ordinary animal instincts.

There is one other reason why the behavioural science of the Skinner box-like model can never satisfactorily predict the whole of human experience and it is this: our human environment is not fixed. Neither are we static. We do not live in a controlled environment. Our lives are subject to and sometimes enabled by random events. Whenever there is uncertainty in our lives, like any other successful species, we can adapt to it. This adaptation is a potential and unpredictable thing, and anything can happen because of our connection to each other. This is where hope lives.

A life well lived relishes this potential. Rather than fearing danger, we can learn to participate in life, to live courageously and imagine a better life. The random potential of life actually enables recovery. Such was the case for Robert after his tragic encounter with the dead man in the park. Suddenly, he came face to face with the harsh reality of his own death and, in a sense, his identification with the dead man helped Robert to see that he had a life to live. This real and totally unforeseen event could not have happened in a controlled environment – and Robert's response to this event could not have happened in any other species. His response was entirely human and it was this human response as much as anything that unlocked Robert's potential for life.

Our lives are more than a set of instinctual behaviours open to modification by association or reward. Our human experiences are also about the random and the unforeseen. And what is more, our relationships are complex and interconnected. In a very real sense, we are about each other. What we think about each other and our challenges matters, at least as much as the way we behave and how we imagine our life to be. Modern psychotherapists recognized the need to address this human reality in a more meaningful way, and so that is exactly what they did. The modern cognitive behavioural movement set about filling this 'holistic gap' in the therapeutic world and, as we shall see, their efforts took us in a whole new and more complete therapeutic direction.

Arthur

ARTHUR IS A FIFTY-YEAR-OLD civil servant. He is diabetic and morbidly obese. He is married to Kate and has two daughters. He became severely depressed after experiencing a prolonged period of bullying at work. This experience resulted in his suspension and a subsequent further catastrophic decline in his mood. At this low point he attempted unsuccessfully to take his own life.

He was referred to my clinic by his GP. In her letter to me she wrote, 'Arthur blames himself for everything. I fear he may be close to the stage where he believes that his death would be a welcome event for everyone.'

Arthur's Initial Assessment

At our first meeting Arthur's attitude was downcast, resigned and reproachful. Not only was he experiencing mental health difficulties – his GP had described him as 'clinically depressed' – but he was also physically unwell. He was self-critical of his attempts at recovery but at this stage he wondered where else he could go from here.

Arthur had a recent history of suicidal behaviour. As is so often the case, he was ambivalent about coming to a mental health assessment. Many others were concerned about him: both his wife and his employers were appealing to him to get help.

At Arthur's first meeting it was clear that he was unwell, but it was not until our meetings progressed that the extent of his physical illness and mental health difficulty became truly apparent. Health problems are multilayered and sometimes they are revealed in slow steps. They emerge like the peeling of a fruit, slowly, to expose the soft flesh underneath or the hard stone of a seed at their centre. They may be as encrusted as the hull of an old barge. Each emotional coating is vital to the whole voyage and so the process of peeling back and considering each layer can be as surprising as it is restorative.

Guilt and self-reproach are destructive human emotions and they are commonly seen in those who struggle to feel well again. Excessive self-criticism is characteristic of people with a long history of anxiety, depression and substance misuse. Shame may be a real problem in these circumstances and its hostile judgements are most destructive to those less able to generate inner feelings of warmth and self-regard.[1] There are times when we all need to be able to soothe ourselves, not just to be reassured by others. Harsh self-criticism is a deeply unpleasant sentiment. Its endurance is incompatible with a well-lived life. Arthur felt shame at sharing his experience with me; it was as though he felt he did not deserve to be listened to.

To live life well we need to be able, and as often as possible, to be good to ourselves. Self-nurturing is a continuing process, so to be well we need to like ourselves. In depression this self-esteem is typically lost and so to recover we need to learn to like ourselves once again.

Unfortunately, once a harsh inner voice takes root in the mind, like it had in Arthur's case, it hardens over time. If it becomes dominant it provides a very depressing commentary. Persistent self-reproach such as this is a challenge to the mentally distressed and to those in recovery. One might ask where such a harsh inner voice could have come from; perhaps from our genes or our past, or our experience of conditioning and learning. Sometimes it is helpful to look back on our childhood in search of a likely origin for our shame. If we look back, we may find scarce experience of warmth or kindness. Self-critical adults tend to judge themselves harshly, just as they were judged harshly in their youth.

---

[1] Paul Gilbert and Sue Procter, 'Compassionate mind training for people with high shame and self-criticism: Overview and pilot study of a group therapy approach', *Clinical Psychology and Psychotherapy*, Vol. 13, 2006, pp. 353–79.

Every life has its setbacks and disappointments. Things must go wrong for each one of us. But when the self-critical fail, what they fear most of all is the shame of their failure.

Shame is trans-diagnostic. As we saw earlier, modern therapists are particularly interested in trans-diagnostic feelings, fears and emotions since they often tell us more about why some women and men find it so difficult to engage with therapy, and why some people find recovery so difficult.

Shame is a disabling human emotion. To overcome its paralysis, we must learn to be more compassionate with ourselves and with others. To recover we need to stop blaming ourselves. Over time in therapy we recognize these painful emotions for what they are and learn to understand how they developed: as defensive strategies protecting us from our most critical fears. From the notes available to me, it was clear that Arthur was a man in grave need of a more compassionate mind.

After discussion with the multidisciplinary team we felt it would be most useful to meet Arthur and suggest a treatment called Compassion Focused Therapy (CFT). Of all the modern therapies described in this book, this has to be one of my favourites. So what is CFT and how is it different from traditional Cognitive Behavioural Therapy?

Compassion Focused Therapy (CFT)

Compassion Focused Therapy (CFT) was developed by Dr Paul Gilbert and his colleagues at the Department of Psychology, University of Derby, UK. It is described as a hybrid of CBT developed especially for people with high levels of shame and self-criticism. CFT has deep roots in cognitive neuroscience as well as social, evolutionary and Buddhist psychology. These elements come together in a therapy that rebuilds a sense of connection and attachment in men and women whose mental life is burdened by such feelings.

CFT differs from traditional CBT in a number of ways. CFT does not target negative thoughts or even seek to correct errors of thinking. Instead, like mindfulness, CFT aims to alter a person's whole relationship with themselves. From the recognition of the source of self-critical thoughts, the treatment proceeds by teaching ideas of acceptance, mindfulness and compassion. Then it tests these out in real experience using behavioural practice in real life.

CFT begins with a neuroscientific hypothesis. According to Gilbert, 'People with high levels of shame and self-criticism struggle to feel relieved, reassured or safe.' Gilbert draws from a large body of animal research data to suggest that human beings possess specialized physiological systems underpinning experience of emotions, such as reassurance, safeness and wellbeing. Compassionate systems probably develop in response to healthy early childhood experiences, and in adulthood they respond to the experience of being cared for with self-calming and a sense of wellbeing.

Of course, other physiological systems are also involved in the regulation of our emotions, our mood and anxiety. Most people will be familiar with the threat protection system. This adrenalin-based system underpins our ability to respond rapidly to hazards – to either fight or take flight. Another system is the dopamine-based drive system, which enables us to seek rewards and respond to incentives for food or sex or rank. This activation system is a source of anticipation and pleasure.

Gilbert proposes that a third system exists and he calls this 'the contentment system'. This diffuse cerebral network probably enables living creatures to experience contentment and to feel at peace when they are not under threat and are not striving for rewards. Gilbert hypothesizes that this contentment system is underdeveloped in people with excessive levels of shame and self-criticism.

It's true that our defensive and our drive systems have become dominant in our life. In modern times many of us live in a constant state of stress, bombarded with twenty-four-hour news alerts sounding a constant alarm as we struggle with daily pressures to make ends meet and still consume ever more. It seems that our adrenalin/dopamine-filled consciousness has overwhelmed our contentment system. Actually our 'contentment system' may be the essential natural basis of a life well lived.

Compassionate Mind Training (CMT)

Compassion may be defined as 'a sensitivity to suffering in oneself (as well as in others) combined with a commitment to try to alleviate it'. When the elements of CFT are put together, they form a curriculum known as Compassionate Mind Training, or CMT. The CFT therapist begins with a functional analysis of critical thoughts and behaviours, and uses this to encourage cognitive behavioural exercises likely to develop empathy and acceptance of distress.

The basic idea of CFT is to help someone learn to understand their distress, so they can be gentle and self-soothing at times of setbacks and failure. CFT reframes all self-critical language within an understanding of self-preservation and so-called safety behaviour.

There is no point in being critical of someone for their self-criticism. The tendency to self-criticism is automatic. It is characteristic in some people for a combination of reasons, including evolutionary defences, genes, learning and conditioning. In CMT, this automatic emotion is not seen as needing correction. Self-critical feelings and reactions are not seen as wrong or someone's fault.

CMT aims to replace the automatic tendency to become self-critical with a learned ability to tolerate negative feelings. CFT/CMT does not encourage a submissive acceptance of self-critical feelings. Instead this therapy encourages the growth of 'a compassionate mind'. This is one that sees self-critical feelings as understandable forms of safety behaviour, a retreat from the shame. CFT views these thoughts as totally automatic and rehearsed. It is not about blame.

The aim of CMT is to develop a new self-compassionate insight into how a person arrived at such a hostile mental position and how they did so completely unintentionally. The key is to understand the feelings that are generated by a person's own hostile thought pattern and behaviour. CFT therapy does not attempt to teach any person to reason differently, rather, and more importantly, it aims to help an individual to feel differently.

Our CFT therapist works with a multidisciplinary team in groups using behaviour and cognitive behavioural methods to promote the attributes of compassion (see p. 192). This educational element of CFT helps to build compassionate thinking, acceptance and mindfulness.

Consistent with standard behavioural practice each individual member of the CFT group is encouraged to keep a behavioural diary and to record their self-critical thoughts. Making diaries and self-ratings in this way is an exercise in any Behaviour Therapy or Cognitive Behavioural Therapy programme. It may be instructive to recall situations and events that prompt self-critical thinking. In this way a person's awareness is increased as well as their understanding of how their critical feelings are prompted. Each thought is rated for its frequency, intrusiveness and duration. The response to each thought is also rated for the degree of anger, hostility and distress associated with it. The degree to which someone can distract themselves from a self-critical thought is also measured.

A similar diary and rating is made for compassionate or self-soothing thoughts in order to consider the situations that bring these more positive feelings about. The group meets regularly and gradually progress is made.

Arthur's Journey Begins

Thursday, 9 April 2015

Arthur is a tall man with broad shoulders. When he comes to see me, he is very overweight. As we speak, he experiences moments of anxiety, which seem to be the result of pressure or stress he feels in the context of our meeting.

'Hello, you're very welcome, Arthur. Please come in and have a seat.'

'Thanks, doctor. I asked them at reception what I should call you. The guy said doctor would be fine.'

'Of course, Arthur. Or Jim, if you prefer?'

'No, I'll stick with doctor. It seems better, if that's OK with yourself?'

'Absolutely, Arthur. So tell me, are you happy to be seeing me today?'

'Well, my GP told me to see you. There is a lot going on in my life. She said I could trust you.'

'She's right – you can trust me.'

'Jesus, sorry about all the sweating here, doctor. You can see that I'm not in great shape. I get these sweats when I'm under pressure.'

'Can I turn down the heat for you or get you a glass of water or anything, Arthur?'

'No, no, I'll be all right. It'll pass, it'll pass.'

'Do you feel under a lot of pressure coming to see me today, Arthur?'

'No, no, I'm just – it's just – well, I'm a worried man, doctor.'

'And is there anything specific that is worrying you?'

'Lots! My GP says that I'm clinically depressed, so that's enough, along with the diabetes, my weight, the gastritis and this awful heartburn . . . Sure, I don't need to tell you that I could do with losing three or four stone. I don't think anyone would even notice that off me. Look, my health is a train wreck.'

'It can be difficult for any of us to manage our issues without help, can't it?'

'Well, that's just it. I've been off work for ages now and it seems to me that my health is deteriorating more and more the longer I'm not working. It should be the other way around, shouldn't it?'

'True, but being out of work can bring its own stresses, can't it?'

'Yeah, it was the stress at work that kicked this whole thing off in the first place. Ironic, no?'

'Well . . .'

'You see, it's all my fault anyway. I do have help. I have a wife and two kids, right? I have to support them. I have huge responsibilities. I need to just shift myself back into gear, but I don't feel able. I feel like I'm going backwards.'

'Getting yourself going again can be hard, Arthur.'

'Well, that's true, but you have to get this straight, right from the off. I'm not here for tea and sympathy. I can get that for free elsewhere. I'm not interested in self-pity. To hell with that!'

'Of course, but surely, Arthur, you deserve help – people deserve respect, don't they, whatever the cause of the problems they may have?'

'Respect? For being depressed? Hah! I have only myself to blame. It's such a shame. I'm ashamed to be talking to you now, but I'm also at the end of my rope here. So I see no other option.'

'And is that really where you feel you are, Arthur?'

'Yes. That's where they have left me, my employers, and I'm not proud of that fact either.'

'Why don't we talk about it?'

'Because, look, in the first place I have to soldier on here. In the second place, what I need from you is a kickstart of some sort. I don't go for the psychological guff. I don't believe people should be encouraged to be depressed, you know? Telling us to "lean into it" and all that crap.'

'That's a bit harsh, Arthur, don't you think?'

'Well, it's the way I see it. Mental health discussion is a bit, well, you know – lame.'

'You won't be surprised that I don't see it that way, Arthur, but it is interesting that you do.'

'Well, that's always been my attitude to the whole touchy-feely approach.'

'Like I said, Arthur, why don't we talk about it for a bit since we are here today. It takes effort to come in here.'

'Look, doctor, it's such a long story, you probably don't even want to hear it. Anyway, I thought this would be more straightforward. I'd come in, you'd give me a prescription for something – you know, some happy pills – patch me up and send me back out there again.'

'Well, maybe you deserve a better response than that. Isn't that what I'm here to give you, Arthur?'

'Maybe.'

Arthur looks very pale now and is sweating profusely.

'Arthur, forgive me for saying, but you don't seem to be very well at all. Can I get you anything?'

'Ah, these sweats are worse. It's the diabetes. I took my insulin just before, in your toilets out there, but I haven't eaten. I should have known. I . . . look, doctor, I need something sugary here and fast. It's the hypoglycemia thing. You know, you're a doctor – well, sort of . . .'

'Arthur, you're soaked in sweat. Let me get you some sweet tea. I have some biscuits here, too. Please eat a couple of those while I make you some tea.'

'Yeah, that'll do the trick, doctor. Thanks.'

After a little while Arthur begins to feel better and he becomes less irritable.

'You look a little better there now, Arthur. Are you OK?'

'Yeah, I just needed the sugar.'

'Whatever about the sympathy, you got the tea anyway!'

'Ha! Yeah, doc, you might be good for something yet.'

'Arthur, if you feel up to it, can we talk some more?'

'Yeah, I'm OK now. I'm good now.'

'So, you do feel better?'

'Yeah, I've been trying so hard to keep a tighter control on the diabetes recently, but I can't even manage that. I should always carry something sweet on me for times like this. But no, I've failed again.'

'Arthur, why did you come here to see me today?'

'I don't know. Like I said, the doctor said, end of my rope. I don't have a clue.'

'But you have come, so why don't we talk about it?'

'Well, like I said, in the first place this is not my style.'

'What's not?'

'This!'

'What's this?'

'Baring my soul to a trick-cyclist! Looking for sympathy.'

'And in the second place?'

'I'm running out of options here, doctor. I mean look at the state of me. I couldn't even shave today! I was never like this. I had pride in my appearance.'

'So why don't we talk?'

'Look, doctor, I feel like, well, like a soldier and I am on the Eastern Front, you know?'

'That must be a very distressing feeling, Arthur.'

'You know they used to write L.M.F on the discharge papers of the soldiers who took the handy way out. L.M.F. – 'Lacks Moral Fibre'. You know it's a century since the Somme. Soldiering is in my background. My dad was a soldier. I've been thinking about all that recently.'

'Is that how you feel about yourself at the moment – L.M.F. – Arthur?'

'Yes, I suppose it is. And so I don't know what it is exactly you could do for me.'

'Maybe if we talk about your health problems, Arthur, it might help us to understand some more about the pressures you have been experiencing.'

'How can talking really help someone like me? Look at the state of me.'

'Yes, but if we make a start . . . It's not just talking for talking's sake. If we try to understand, then maybe we could learn to make some changes.'

'Like what changes?'

'Well, we don't know yet. But one thing is clear to me, Arthur, you could have better health and a better life. You have to believe that, don't you?'

'Hmm.'

'Arthur, you said to me earlier that you were trying so hard. That's true, isn't it?'

'Yes, it's true. But, doc, there are no marks for effort in this life. Results are all that count at the end of the day. My father used to say that to me – often.'

'Actually, effort does matter, Arthur. It has to matter. We need to reward our efforts.'

'See, there you are, out with the pity straight away! God loves a trier! Doc, give me a break!'

'No, Arthur. I'm not pitying you. What I'm saying is that, to me, you seem to be a very brave man. Definitely not Lacking Moral Fibre. Not a coward. Not at all. You have to have great courage to deal with what's on your plate.'

'I haven't told you the half of it.'

'Right, then think about it. Your stress, your diabetes, your depression – they are all real, aren't they? You didn't just make them up, did you?'

'No, I did not. These things are real. I sure do feel them.'

'Arthur, your health is about the whole of your life, right?'

'Yeah, but why would I talk to a shrink about my general health? Are you qualified for that as well?'

'Yes, I'm a psychiatrist, but that is to say I am a medical doctor who specializes in the mind as well as the body. The two go together, you know? I work with many other health professionals, including nurses and physicians and psychologists. We're a team.'

'Good for you! But when all's said and done the stuff in my head is not going to be helped by a load of kind words from you or your team.'

'But it could be – and maybe it's urgent now. Mental health problems make physical health problems worse. Your entire health could become a matter of life and death.'

'Thanks for that, very reassuring. Christ!'

'Forgive me, Arthur.'

'Look, it's OK, that's the usual sort of stuff you guys always say. But I'm not part of your world.'

'*My world*, Arthur? What world?'

'Your "mental" world. I live in the real world. It's dog-eat-dog out there. Just see how far kind words will get you when you can't pay your bloody mortgage. Do you realize that my wife had to go back to work to help out with the bills? Can you imagine how that makes me feel?'

'I see it distresses you, Arthur. It's clear that you are very critical of yourself.'

'What difference does that make?'

'It could be the basis for a whole new approach to your difficulties.'

'I told you, I'm not up for some psychobabble.'

'Your GP is very concerned about you, Arthur.'

'I suppose she told you that I was suicidal, did she?'

'Yes, she did.'

'Well, let's get this straight. I'm not, OK? I'm not suicidal. You can call off the men in the white coats. You needn't worry, I'm not going to kill myself.'

'But was there ever a time when you were suicidal, Arthur?'

'Yeah, I have been, in the past. I even took an overdose, once, before, made a complete mess of that, and if a bus had hit me crossing Thomas Street some evening I don't think I would have minded. But now I know I have my responsibilities. I have to provide for my wife and kids. They need me. So my life's not in danger – not from suicide, anyway.'

'Good. But Arthur, let's talk about things anyway. Let's talk about a combined approach to the whole of your health.'

'Look, doctor, I have to go. I have to pick something up in town for my wife, Kate. She's working this evening.'

'Would you consider coming back to see me again, Arthur, so we can continue our conversation?'

'Really, doctor, what is there to talk about?'

'You and your health, and why you're so critical about yourself, and how we can help you to feel a whole lot better. How about having that conversation?'

'That's a big agenda, doc!'

'It's worth talking about, surely.'

'I could do with feeling better. I just don't see how talking will do that for me.'

'It could do. I don't suppose you have ever heard of a therapy called Compassion Focused Therapy, or CFT?'

'Doc, is there no end to it? CFT! Whatever will they think of next. I suppose it's like I said, God loves a trier.'

'Will you think about it, Arthur? About CFT?'

'CFT, eh? I haven't a clue. I will need a bit of time to think about doing therapy.'

'Good. Think about it. You can do no more than that. You're very welcome to come back. Make an appointment any time. In the meantime, I'll write back to your GP to update her, but just give us a call.'

'Well, who knows, maybe I will. But if I come back it's only for the biscuits!'

'At least our biscuits are effective!'

Thursday, 23 April 2015

Arthur returns two weeks later. Although this time he seems in a better physical state, his manner is still sceptical and ambivalent, and he is still blaming himself.

'Well, I came back. I'm not sure why, but I'm here. I guess it's "Paging Dr Freud" time.'

'I'm glad to see you again, Arthur. And it's good you came back. I had hoped you would.'

'Yeah, well, you know I really hate this stuff. It's just I don't deserve this. I'm just not any good at it.'

'Not any good at what, Arthur?'

'You know, talking about myself. I don't believe in giving myself that kind of space. It's not in my nature. It's painful.'

'Arthur, would you mind if I made an observation?'

'Go ahead, doctor. Open fire.'

'Well, it seems to me that you are extremely hard on yourself.'

'Yeah, so?'

'Can we try to imagine that you had a less critical voice? That you could maybe develop a kinder voice for yourself?'

'Are you saying I am not kind? Well, I can be kind, and caring. I'm caring towards my children, that comes easy to me. I'm kind to my wife.'

'But it seems to me that it is much less easy for you to be kind to yourself.'

'Well, of course. It's easy for me to be kind and caring towards my kids – they're so innocent.'

'And you're not? What crime are you guilty of?'

'None, I suppose. Except I am always, you know, I'm constantly on guard – hyperaware, all the time.'

'What do you think is going to happen?'

'Anything, really. It's a very hard world out there. And I have to protect my family. I'm always telling them to be careful.'

'So you might say that you feel there is danger at every turn?'

'Yeah, there could be, you never know.'

'What do you fear most?'

'Who knows? Getting it wrong, my own stupidity, I don't know how to put it . . . I suppose it's the judgement of others.'

'And so you judge yourself harder than anyone?'

'Ironic, eh?'

'Arthur, do you ever think about taking some time to relax, time to be at ease, so to speak?'

'Relax?'

'That's right. Taking some time to laugh, even at yourself.'

'So now you're telling me I'm ridiculous! Seriously?'

'No, Arthur, I'm not saying that. I'm not saying that at all. I'm saying that you are a very sensitive man.'

'So what if I am?'

There is a pause here as we both re-evaluate where the conversation has taken us.

'Could we maybe talk about your background, Arthur? Your childhood, growing up and—'

'Ah, Jesus, here we go . . . You know, doctor, I have done therapy before.'

'Have you, Arthur?'

'Yeah, a couple of years ago. Does it not say that on my file?'

'No, it doesn't say much about that, Arthur.'

'Well, I did. CBT. Yeah, nice fella. He did his best, I have to say, but it didn't do anything much for me. About four sessions – I knocked it on the head after that.'

'Did you take anything from it, Arthur?'

'A few things, I suppose.'

'Like what? Do you remember any of them?'

'Eh, I do remember the guy telling me that therapy was not all about looking back.'

'That's true – well, actually it depends.'

'Yeah, he used to say it was best to stay in the here and now. But then he also used to say that shame and guilt have deep roots. Come to think of it, I do remember those little nuggets.'

'I think you're right there, Arthur. It's about an assessment. Each person in distress has their own individual needs. Sometimes we need to understand the past. Everyone has different issues, so the same rules needn't apply. One size does not fit all.'

'Sounds a bit random to me.'

'Can I talk to you about something else entirely, Arthur?'

'Go ahead.'

'Do you like gardening, Arthur?'

'Now I'm definitely not sure where this is going, doctor, but go ahead.'

'Think of it like this: let's say your mind is a garden and you want to look after it as best you can, OK?'

'OK.'

'So sometimes you mow the grass, sometimes you sweep the leaves, but sometimes you need to dig a little. Sometimes you need to dig up old roots.'

'Well, actually I was never one for the gardening, doctor. I'll leave that to your man on the radio, what's-his-face . . .'

'OK, but if you would just humour me, Arthur. Let's just think about it for a moment.'

'OK, go on.'

'Suppose we could understand the past, then maybe we could find out where the old roots lie. We could dig them up and clear them from the garden and that could help with the present. What do you think?'

'Gardening lessons from a shrink? Christ, I've heard it all now.'

'What do you say, Arthur? Would you be willing to maybe talk about it?'

'And what could I learn from digging up old ground?'

'Maybe in that old ground we might find some old roots that need digging up. You told me last time we met, Arthur, that you felt ashamed being here talking to me.'

'Yeah.'

'Why do you still feel that shame?'

'Well, it's real, isn't it?'

'Yes, of course it's real. But that feeling could be killing you.'

'I think you'll find it's the diabetes and my weight that's killing me, doctor.'

'But if you look at it another way, your shame is toxic as well and nobody is helping you with that issue.'

'You're trying to tell me that shame could kill me? Come on, give me a break.'

'Arthur, maybe in understanding your shame – where it comes from – we could make you feel a lot better.'

'Look, I'll think about it. The coming back to talk to you about my past bit, I mean. I'll think about it, you know.'

'That's good to hear, Arthur. If you did come back, I think we could help you.'

'Yeah, anyway, I'm going to leave it there for today, doctor, if that's OK. I'm sure you've got a waiting room full of wrecks like me to deal with.'

'Not really, Arthur. The people here are just like you and me. You couldn't tell any of us apart in the average queue.'

'I am not so sure. I stick out like a sore thumb and I know I'm the patient!'

'We'll all be patients of some sort or other at some stage in our lives. All of us.'

Thursday, 7 May 2015

When Arthur returns he is more willing to talk. It isn't clear if he will engage in therapy, but at least he has come back and so that is a start.

'You see, doctor, nothing I did was ever good enough for him. Nothing.'

'You said your father was an army man, is that right?'

'Yes, he was. 24/7. Being in the army is not like other professions. Or it wasn't for him anyway. He didn't clock off at five. He brought the army back home, evenings and weekends.'

'So I take it that he was never out of uniform, so to speak?'

'That's for sure. He was one tough monkey, I can tell you. And you know the weird thing?'

'What's that?'

'There was nothing more in this world I wanted than to follow him into the army.'

'But you didn't, did you?'

'No, I failed the medical. Three bloody times!'

'Were you unwell, Arthur?'

'No, I wasn't unwell. It was my hearing, would you believe? I've had a slight problem with my left ear since I was a kid. It's really nothing, but it was enough for me to fail the medical. I was absolutely gutted, you know?'

'And was your father still alive at that time in your life?'

'Yeah. He said nothing when I told him. Nothing at all. Like he didn't hear what I was saying. Like I wasn't even there.'

'That's tough on a young man, Arthur. He gave you the silent treatment?'

'I knew what he was thinking, though. "Not good enough. My son, the failure, let me down again."'

'Wow, those are harsh words, Arthur.'

'Well, he didn't actually say them, but I knew that's what he thought. I could tell.'

'Were you under a lot of pressure to succeed?'

'From my father? Yes, very much so. He was always judging me, rating me.'

'Silently?'

'Yeah, he wouldn't say much, but nothing was good enough – and I could tell when he wasn't impressed.'

'And your mother?'

'Ah, my mother was different. She was English by birth, you know? They were an unusual match-up for that time in Ireland. My father was quite the nationalist, but he married an English woman.'

'And what did your mother do?'

'She was a nurse. She was a kind woman, for sure.'

'What do you think they wanted you to achieve, your parents?'

'That's just it. I never knew. They never said.'

'Are they still alive today?'

'No, they're long gone now. Nearly twenty years. Our girls were only small at the time. My father passed away first. My mother didn't last long after him.'

'Would you say that they were very strict?'

'The atmosphere in our house was always tense. Well, when my father was around anyway, there was a real feeling of . . . well, walking on eggshells is the best way to describe it. He wasn't easy to live with.'

'You had to walk on tiptoe around him?'

'Yes, and my mother felt that way too. I know she did. He was a fearsome man.'

'Was he ever physically violent with you or your mother?'

'No, not that I saw. Just relentlessly critical and opinionated.'

'Do you have any memories of affection from your parents?'

'There were certainly no kisses and hugs, if that's what you mean, but I did feel a bond with my mother.'

'In what way?'

'I sometimes imagined it like we were in the trenches together – a team, on constant alert, ready at a moment's notice, as if something awful could happen at any minute.'

'So you learned to live with the jeopardy?'

'Yeah, you could say that.'

'And when something *bad* would happen, how would it make you feel?'

'I'd feel it was all my fault.'

'But you were just a boy?'

'Yeah, but there was no one else to blame.'

'You know that you weren't really to blame, don't you?'

'That's just it. I don't know. But if I wasn't, then neither was my mother. "Just keep your head down, Arty," she'd say to me, sort of quietly, under her breath.'

'And that's what you did?'

'Absolutely. But not any more.'

'Not any more? How so?'

'I get my retaliation in first these days. I don't wait. I strike the first blow.'

'What do you mean, Arthur?'

'Well, I blame myself because I have a situation at work. It's the reason I'm on a sabbatical. That's what I'm telling anyone who asks. It's gardening leave, as they say.'

'Tell me about it, Arthur.'

'Is there much point?'

'Yes, there is. I am still hoping to enrol you in our therapy. Do you remember, it's called CFT – Compassion Focused Therapy? You'd like it. I work with a CFT therapist. Her name is Irene. In fact, I'd like you to meet. She runs a CFT group and together they all learn how to have more compassionate minds.'

'Sounds like a mouthful to me.'

'Would you be willing to meet Irene and—'

'Learn to be compassionate to her?'

'No, Arthur, learn to be compassionate to yourself.'

'Sure, that would be nice!'

Thursday, 21 May 2015

Arthur had begun to attend our CFT group and after his first few sessions he comes back for a review. This time he remains his usual self-critical, sceptical self.

'I've met your Irene! She is very impressive.'

'Arthur, just for the record, she's not my Irene. Maybe she is our Irene?'

'Yeah, whatever. Actually, she says she can help me, so thank you for asking me to see her.'

'You talked to her about your problems?'

'A little.'

'Tell me.'

'What do you want to know?'

'About you and your life, maybe?'

'I'm a civil servant. I work in a government department. I'm here to serve the people, the people of Ireland, to the best of my ability. I take my work very seriously. I love my country. Actually, that's why I have been suspended.'

'Oh? It is a responsible job.'

'Absolutely. That's why I couldn't just stand by and say nothing about what was going on. Someone had to stand up and blow the whistle.'

'And that person was you?'

'Sure, I felt like that little boy in the fairy story – you know the one, 'The Emperor's New Clothes'. I felt it was my duty to do something.'

'You feel very passionately about this, Arthur.'

'You're damn right I do. This has been my battle, for the good of the country. That's the way I see it.'

'And did your standing up and blowing the whistle resolve your difficulties in work?'

'Not at all. That was just the start of it. I had absolutely no desire to be unpopular – I prefer to be well-liked – but that's just not what happens in these situations.'

'Did you have any support from your colleagues?'

'Christ, no. I was left standing all alone. That's what sickens me the most. The message from my colleagues was: "Keep your head down, knuckle under, don't rock the boat or you'll drag us all down with you."'

'This was around the time of the financial crash, the end of the Celtic Tiger?'

'Yeah, the Celtic Tiger! Jesus, give me a break. You see, I could see that the sums didn't add up. It was clear as day to me! I knew well that the tiger was just about to turn around and bite us in the arse. Big time!'

'So what did you do?'

'Well, no one would listen to me. No one respected my opinion. I am not an economist. They were just ignoring me, like I was stupid. So I took action.'

'And that rattled a few cages, I'm guessing?'

'That's the understatement of the year.'

Thursday, 28 May 2015

When Arthur returns the following week, he is very downcast. We begin by talking about his mood. He starts to describe his depression to me.

'Just . . . dread. That's the only way I can describe it. I wake up early. And when I say wake up I mean, like, I don't sleep, barely a wink.'

'And do you dread the coming day, Arthur?'

'Yes, every minute of it. It's like I'm just waiting to die – the dread of that. Can you imagine?'

'It's hard to imagine, Arthur.'

'I'm just empty, you know? Completely void of energy and this is before I even get out of the bloody bed! Sometimes I wish the ground would just open up and swallow me.'

'And do you feel your mood is any better or worse at the end of the day?'

'How do you mean?'

'Well, is there any pattern to your mood?'

'Not really. It doesn't get better anyway. I long for sleep at the end of the day, but . . .'

'You say that you're empty, Arthur.'

'Yeah, empty, like I'm all out of fuel. My energy is shot. I used to be so full of life. Any of the joy I had left has been replaced with . . . well, dread, you know?'

'Can you enjoy anything?'

'Not any more. It's as though my sense of humour just got up and died. I can't remember the last time I really laughed. My bones ache. They actually ache. Real pain. I'm not imagining it, you know.'

'I believe you, Arthur. Can I ask you something personal?'

'Go ahead. At this stage I have thrown caution to the wind!'

'Tell me, Arthur, do you care about your own wellbeing?'

'What do you mean?'

'Do you want to live well?'

'Of course I do. Sure I wouldn't be here if I didn't.'

'Well, that's good. Irene tells me you have been going to the CFT group.'

'Yeah, but I just feel like, Jesus, I just think, will I ever be right? Am I ever going to be well again?'

'Arthur, let me assure you, I believe that you will be well. It's clear to me that you are very depressed, it's real suffering. But it will get better.'

'But when? How?'

'The CFT can help. It's about your care and gaining a more compassionate mind.'

'Irene's telling me that I can learn to think differently. Do you really think so?'

'Yes, and you can also feel differently as well. We're both certain you can. Your mind needs to be less condemning, less . . . critical of yourself, and this would make space for your mood – or your spirits, if you like – to rise.'

'Is that so? Well, let me ask you a question. Why do you care anyway? Why would you give a toss about someone like me?'

'Arthur, I'm here to care about your wellbeing, that's what I do.'

'Sounds like an odd way to make a living.'

'Not that odd at all, actually. Lots of people care.'

'So are you and Irene just naturally sympathetic – or did you just do a course or something?'

'It takes a bit more than that. Basic sympathy requires very little effort, you know?'

'Yeah, well, you know my feelings on sympathy, doctor.'

'However it takes real effort to try and imagine how someone is feeling – to be empathetic, to try to understand their inner world.'

'You want to get inside my head?'

'Well, yes, in a way. We can both get inside your head, as you put it. Suppose for a second, Arthur, you could develop the skills of compassion and an especially useful skill, "empathy for yourself", if you like.'

'I don't know if someone like me could do that, though.'

'You might, and then you could become more forgiving of yourself, less condemning, less critical. You know, you might have less shame, Arthur.'

'But I don't have any room for self-pity. I told you. Are you listening at all over there?'

'Yes, I did hear you, but what you call "room for self-pity" could actually be room for something entirely different.'

'Like what?'

'Let's try to remember a time when you were kind to yourself and others were also kind to you in return. Can you remember such a time?'

'My wife, Kate, is kind. I am trying to listen to her kindness towards me and respond in a different way – not just dismiss it as pity – but it's not easy.'

'Kate's kindness makes for sharp contrast to the behaviour you have been experiencing at work, I take it?'

'I guess so. Would you believe that it only dawned on me recently that I was being bullied? All along I was the weak one, being bullied. I could never imagine myself as the weak one.'

'But then you responded to them?'

'Yeah, I suppose. It's so embarrassing, though, the things they used to do to me.'

'Tell me what they did.'

'Well, some of it was just so childish; infantile, in fact. These people had responsible jobs, and they're bringing in empty sweet wrappers from home and filling my wastepaper bin with them. It was a great source of amusement for them. Bunch of assholes.'

'That was cruel, Arthur.'

'You know, doctor, it's an awful thing, being fat, you know that? You go from being respected, professional, all that, to just being "that tub of lard" – lard! I have never once commented on the physical appearance of a peer but you get overweight and all of a sudden it's open season. People see you as fair game, like kids ganging up on the weak one. It just strangles your soul.'

'Sounds like a toxic working environment.'

'Yeah, a few smart-arses from the office – you know, the open-plan-type offices – would walk up to my desk with their lunches and just stand there eating in front of me. All to a chorus of sniggers around the place. Pathetic.'

'Was it just your appearance that they targeted?'

'No, there was much worse than that. You know I have poor hearing in my left ear, well anyway, they would purposely turn down the ringer on my phone when I went away from my desk. Did they really think I was that stupid that I wouldn't notice?'

'But you took them on?'

'I did, but then things took a different turn.'

'What happened?'

'I was missing important meetings because I wasn't being included on the memos about them – purposefully – and my superiors started to get on to me about this. They were getting very annoyed about it.'

'And could you explain to any of them what was going on?'

'No, sure, they knew well!'

'Had you no support?'

'No, that's when I felt I had to do something.'

'So what did you do?'

'You see, from time to time I'd be asked to deal with material for the freedom of information act: requests for written answers to parliamentary questions, press releases, all sensitive stuff. You know the kind of response that is expected. All's well with the government, blah, blah, we're on budget, we're on target, nothing to see here, folks, so move along now please, that sort of crap. So this was my opportunity to get something going here.'

'How so?'

'Well, I was able to bury some information in all the usual bull that told it like it really was. I mean not the way they wanted it to look. Then it went out unaltered and someone spotted it and ran with the story. Boom!'

'Wow! I take it that they were not best pleased with you, Arthur?'

'Shit hitting a fan wouldn't do this justice. I may not have a PhD, I may not be a qualified economist, but I know what I'm talking about. My supervisor went berserk, out of control like. She threatened to have me dismissed, then and there. But luckily I'm a civil servant in Ireland, so lots of luck with that.'

'But there were consequences for your employment?'

'Yeah, after a few more stand-up rows I found myself on gardening leave with no end in sight. Actually my GP has signed me off as being unable to attend work. I don't regret it, though, not for a second. I'd do it in a heartbeat again. My best day's work ever. You can't argue with the truth, you know?'

'So you didn't back down.'

'No. It's still in the courts now. Of course they've got the best lawmen on the job, no budget problems there. It's been really rough on me and Kate, and the kids. Imagine, their dad out of work, looking like some kind of layabout.'

'Do you have other options, choices, Arthur?'

'No way. I'm fighting them to the bitter end. Once I'd started down that road, I wasn't for turning, not me.'

'Arthur, would you mind answering a direct question?'

'Go on.'

'Do you think perhaps a more politically savvy-minded way to deal with this work situation would be to duck and dive, stay out of trouble at work, live to fight another day?'

'This has absolutely nothing to do with politics. I blew the whistle. It was the right thing to do. To me the whistle-blowers are the heroes of modern Ireland.'

'So then you took the overdose?'

'Yeah, not too long after that, yeah. The overdose.'

The Six Attributes and Six Skills of Compassion

The methods Irene uses in her group sessions promote awareness and understanding. She uses behaviour examples to test out ideas of acceptance and distress tolerance in daily life, and works with the members of the group to promote an awareness of the six attributes of compassion. These are described in CFT as:

- Care for wellbeing
- Sensitivity
- Sympathy
- Tolerance of distress
- Empathy
- Non-judgement

The CFT therapist encourages the growth of these attributes by teaching the six skills of compassion. These are:

- Compassionate attention
- Reasoning
- Behaviour
- Imagery
- Feeling
- Sensation

A typical CFT group session with Irene involves talking and listening, as well as a review of ongoing cognitive behavioural exercises.

According to Dr Paul Gilbert, the best analogy for CFT therapy might be to consider it a kind of mental physiotherapy. In that way CFT can be seen as a method of promoting the growth of new emotional muscles. The aim of CFT is to teach each individual to create within themselves many more compassionate feelings of warmth, kindness and support. This therapy may be done more easily in a group atmosphere, where the human fellowship emphasizes kindness, common humanity and mindfulness.

Also according to Gilbert, 'It is common for people with high shame and self-criticism, particularly those from harsh backgrounds, to find that the first experience of compassionate therapy, of warmth and kindness, ignites within them considerable sadness and grief.' This is what he calls the 'distress call of the defensive system': it is calling the person to move away from the experience of being cared for. This is actually the moment when CFT therapy really begins to take effect. It is the opportunity for the therapist and the individual to work together to accept and validate their critical feelings.

It is also a mindful moment, to be experienced in the present, when each individual has the opportunity to experience a new way of living and to choose to live life well. The CFT group helps individuals to see self-blame as an unhelpful but understandable defence mechanism. CFT uses compassionate mind training to show how each aspect of self-criticism has some functional aspect behind it and is usually self-defensive. With CFT, Arthur learns to be compassionate about this too.

Thursday, 4 June 2015

Arthur comes to his next session with me after another group meeting. He is keen to discuss his progress.

'I told Irene about the overdose. It came up in the group.'
    'What did you say about it?'
    'It failed, obviously.'
    'You regret you survived?'
    'No, not now. Now it scares me, though. It might have worked

– one more pill, who knows? But I am ashamed of what I did.'

'So you do regret taking the overdose?'

'It's not a question of regret. It wasn't an impulsive act, if that's what you mean.'

'Explain that to me, Arthur.'

'At that time I had lost all hope. I just wanted to lie down and die. Depression is like having tunnel vision. You can't see any other way out.'

'And what about your family – were they affected?'

'They were suffering because of me. I hated that fact. I hated myself for that, but I couldn't let this thing at work go. It was all I had left to hang on to. You have to understand that, doctor.'

'Yes, Arthur, I do. It was a terrible situation to find yourself in.'

'I couldn't sleep, I couldn't work, I couldn't win, I couldn't do anything – but most of all I still couldn't let it go! I just . . .'

'You just lost hope?'

'My GP had me on the happy pills at that stage. She had really been giving me grief about my general health, you know, the weight and all that. I was in a bad way. My world was closing in on me, I had to do something.'

'And that something was to take an overdose of your pills?'

'Yes. I felt at the time that I had to take action, do something for me and my family, you know – stand up and be counted. And I thought, well, this will really stick it to them at work. How are they going to feel now? That thought actually crossed my mind!'

'Actually, you were injuring yourself.'

'I poured the whole bloody bottle of pills down my neck and took a couple of painkillers to boot. My hands were shaking violently, my whole body. All that was in the fridge to get them down with was a sodding carton of juice. It's the last thing I remember before I passed out, the smiley face on that poxy carton of orange juice.'

'But someone called the emergency services?'

'Yeah, I was out of the hospital after a couple of days. The shame when the girls realized what I had done, and Kate, and bloody nosy neighbours. I just don't know. I felt like, *How the hell did I get here?*'

'You must have been under so much pressure, Arthur.'

'I thought at the time – well, I was going to die soon anyway, with the diabetes and the weight and the stress. I was being pushed over the cliff, so maybe I could take charge of the situation, you know. Go out on my terms.'

'And now, Arthur, how do you feel today?'

'About the suicide?'

'About life in general?'

'Look, I'm not great, as you know, but I'm not down there. I'm up here, seeing you, going to the group. Learning all this stuff about the attributes of compassion!'

'Yes, and I'm glad you are here, Arthur, and I'm sure your family is so relieved that you were found in time.'

Compassionate Imagery

One interesting technique in CFT is the use of compassionate imagery as part of compassionate mind training. Here the therapist invites each person to imagine their ideal image of caring and compassion. The use of such imagery is a long-established feature of Buddhist meditation and mindful practice. The ideal image can have qualities of wisdom, strength and warmth. It is an image of non-judgemental acceptance and this is perceived by the individual as warm. An image such as this may be the ideal or perfect nurturer. Each person in the CFT group is encouraged to generate such an image or a number of images for himself or herself.

Thursday, 18 June 2015

Arthur's task at the CFT group was to conjure up a compassionate image and imagine how it might feel or act with him. He explains his thought process.

'You know, doctor, Irene asks us to imagine things. How strange is that? I thought you went to a "shrink" *because* you were imagining things!'

'She probably asked you to imagine something kind, Arthur.'

'Yes, that's it, and at first, you know, I couldn't really do it, but then I sort of got into it. I'm not sure why. All I could imagine was rice pudding! I mean, the warm creamy kind that fills your tummy. I suppose I didn't put this weight on for nothing! The others were imagining a tropical beach on a desert island, but all I could think of was milk pudding!'

'It's a warm image, it could work.'

'Then I was thinking, why have I thought of that?'

'And do you know now?'

'I imagine it's about my granny. She was my dad's mother. I never told you about her. She was musical and she got me playing the guitar. I stopped doing that years ago, but I was good back then.'

'What was your granny like?'

'She was the one really kind and generous person in my childhood. I remember how she told us, my mother and me, to pay no attention to her son, my dad.'

'What would she do?'

'She would feed us. Chicken soup was always on the range and best of all was rice pudding in a bowl with the toasted skin on top.'

'Ambrosia?'

'Yes, heavenly! For a kid, it was magical comfort.'

'And what would Granny say to you now?'

'I imagine she would tell us it's going to be all right!'

'Granny rice is a good image.'

'It's nice to think of her.'

'Arthur, let's imagine how her kindness and wisdom might help you now.'

Thursday, 2 July 2015

Arthur comes back to see me. He still has much to talk about.

'Look, I am so ashamed of what I did. It was the wave of depression that nearly swept me away, when I think of the consequences for Kate and the girls. Look, doctor, I want to get as far away as I possibly can from that place, do you understand me?'

'Absolutely, Arthur.'

'I hope so. Christ, do I hope so.'

'Arthur, after everything you've been through, would you not just consider maybe settling with your employers?'

'Oh, you are fuckin' joking me now! What? I don't believe this! Settle? Settle! Are you out of your mind? Christ! Are you really saying this to me now?'

'Please, Arthur. Please, have a seat . . . Please sit back down and we can discuss this.'

'Don't tell me to compromise. Not now – not after everything I've been through. Do not tell me to take the blame!'

'Arthur, you need to calm down and come and sit down over here with me. Try to relax. OK? Let's take a minute here to just take a breath and discuss this calmly. We can do that, can't we?'

'You talk about having some sort of "plan" for my recovery? Well, I can tell you right here and now, if that plan involves my surrender I'm not doing it. No way! Imagine if they were to get away with it and I took the blame? What sort of a country would we – what sort of life would that be?'

'Look, Arthur, it's certainly not in my plan to upset you. These are all decisions that you will make yourself. No one is forcing you. Least of all me. Anyway, let's just park that idea.'

'Yeah, let's. I have to say, doctor, it's not one of your better ideas, you know?'

'OK, Arthur. Point taken. Shall we talk about something else? Maybe about your family some more?'

'I thought we'd been through all that?'

'I mean your wife and children. We haven't talked about them much.'

'Well, there is not much to say except they are the centre of my world. They mean everything to me and I know I've been letting them down.'

'What do you mean?'

'Kate has had to go back to work to help cover the bills. My sick pay is not covering me enough. And the girls? Well, they are both working now too, but they still need their dad.'

'Could I suggest something, Arthur? Maybe Kate would like to come along to our next session. How would you feel about that?'

'I suppose . . . I'd have no problem with it, I think. She'd have to want to come, though. I can't make her.'

Thursday, 16 July 2015

At our next meeting Arthur comes accompanied by his wife, Kate. She is youthful, smiling and smartly dressed. Arthur introduces her to me and we shake hands.

'This is Kate, my wife, doctor.'

'Great to meet you, Kate. Take a seat, please. Thank you for coming. Would you like a glass of water or anything?'

'I told her about your biscuits.'

'Oh good, good. Would you like one, Kate?'

'Don't mind him, doctor. He's just being a smart-arse!'

'Oh, OK, well if you ever change your mind, I've got some nice chocolate ones. Just recently stocked up!'

'Thanks, but I'm fine for the minute, doctor.'

'So, where should we start today?'

'You tell me, doctor.'

'OK, Arthur. Maybe we could start with you, Kate. Are you happy to be here with us today?'

'Yeah, no problem with me. I wanted to come. I've come here for Arthur. We're all concerned for him, me and the girls – we have two daughters, you know?'

'Yes, Arthur told me.'

'Well, they're both worried about their dad, naturally enough.'

'I see, so Arthur, are you happy for us to talk together, openly, today?'

'Kate can say whatever she likes. I've never been the boss of her, isn't that right, love?'

'Ah, go on. I don't know about that!'

'Is there anything in particular you'd like to say, Kate?'

'Look, I think that Arthur is the one who needs to talk. I know him better than anyone. We are a close-knit family, no secrets or lies.'

'That's right, we are.'

'Yeah, and Arthur is a man of principles. I've always admired him for that. But he has taken this thing so much to heart, doctor.'

'In what way, Kate?'

'Well, his problems have consumed him. I think, anyway.'

'And how has this affected you, Kate?'

'It is starting to take over my life, too. And that's not good for me, I know that.'

'And is there anything you feel you can do?'

'I decided to go back out into the working world. Me sitting around all day looking at him looking at me was not producing any results, let me tell you.'

'Well, we needed the extra pay cheque too, doctor.'

'Arthur, that's not true. How many times have we discussed this? Your sick pay is fine, a few minor cutbacks and we'd happily survive on it, you know that. This sacrifice stuff is all in your head. This "You had to go back to work because we needed the money." Rubbish! It's not true! Sorry, doctor.'

'But, the girls, Kate, they need me to provide for—'

'Arthur, come on! The girls are fine. They're earning, probably more than us at this stage. They're clever, and well qualified, and they can look after themselves. They are very self-sufficient girls, doctor, you know?'

'Responsible young women!'

'That they are, doctor. I know they'll always be Dad's little girls in his eyes, and that's fine, but they don't need us to support them any more – not financially, anyway.'

'Yeah, but what if there's a wedding or—'

'Arthur, will you stop? The point is, doctor, that financially we are fine. Of course you could always find room for a little more, but we're fine. And it's been a release for me going back to work, I'm just loving it.'

'And what is it that you work at, Kate?'

'Well, it's only part time, but my friend's daughter is a florist and I'm doing a few hours there every day. It's nearby and I just love working with flowers and being back out in the world again. It makes a refreshing change.'

'Had you not worked for long, Kate?'

'I was a qualified dental hygienist back in the day, before we had the two girls, and I liked it, but I didn't fancy getting back into all that. Those kinds of jobs change a lot in a few years. And besides, the florist work is just an absolute joy for me. Buying flowers for someone is a wonderful thing to do, you know?'

'Sounds like you're really enjoying your work there, Kate?'

'Totally. I couldn't be happier with that end of things.'

'I still feel the guilt of this, though, doctor.'

'Now, hang on, Arthur. Look, me going back out to work is about me. I have to keep myself well too. You're a great father and a great man, but this endless catastrophic debate has got to come to an end. This thing will be resolved, one way or another! Look, doctor, I want the old happy, funny, loving Arthur back.'

'Arthur is working towards that, Kate. We are all working towards that.'

'I know Arthur needs your help, doctor, and I'm trying desperately to help. But it's like I'm walking on eggshells around him, having to tiptoe around him!'

'Kate, you're making me sound like my father now!'

'Doctor, the overdose frightened the life out of the girls and me. I really didn't see it coming. Yeah, I knew he was under pressure, but – suicide? I was just saying to him a few days before all that: "Do you want to be right – or do you want to be well again?" I didn't know he was so low, I really didn't know. So I also feel guilty about that.'

'You've nothing to be feeling guilty about, darling, nothing at all. I was trying to hide it from you.'

'Yes, but don't you see, I am here today because I want you to be well.'

'You are both here together speaking openly about it now. That's real progress, isn't it, Kate? Don't you think so too, Arthur?'

'Yeah, doctor, and so I would like to do whatever it takes to help Arthur. I'm sure you can see that.'

'Of course, Kate. So, Arthur, during the last session we talked about a recovery plan, among other things.'

'Yeah, doctor, I meant to say that. Look, I'm really sorry about my attitude that day, but you really hit my sensitive spot. It was like the last straw, you know? I really needed to think of Granny's rice pudding for a while after it, to calm myself and see some reason.'

'Arthur told me about imagining Granny's pudding, doctor. I remember his granny. She was a lovely, kind old person when I first knew her.'

'It's good, Kate, to have some image of kindness and wisdom when you're in a panic.'

'Arthur has been telling about seeing Irene and the group and his CFT therapy. I am so glad he is doing a therapy. I never thought he would stick with it, but he has and I am proud of him for that as well!'

'You're right, Kate. Therapy can be difficult, but Arthur has stayed the course this time.'

'And do you know, doctor, I think I have learned a lot. I have to admit I am beating myself up a bit less.'

'So could we talk now, all three of us, about the next phase of your care plan? Are you willing to discuss it now, Arthur?'

'Yes, we are, doctor. Definitely. Aren't we, Arthur?'

'Yeah, Kate, you know I want to be well, so what's the plan?'

'Arthur, the best therapeutic approach is always holistic. That is to say it's about your health and your lifestyle, as well as compassion and acceptance. Your care plan should use a range of methods: psychological, sociological and biological. We like to say here that it's about doing whatever it takes.'

'Jesus, it sounds like heavy stuff, doctor.'

'Not really, Arthur, it's just about the whole of your health. So we want to look again at your physical health as well as your mental health.'

'What are you getting at, doctor?'

'Would you consider coming in to our day service – we call it our Wellness and Recovery Centre. It's a multidisciplinary service, with nursing staff and some GPs, and mindfulness and fitness all combined. You could be there with Irene and the rest of the team to get your mental and physical health back on track.'

'I suppose I am still not really sure what this involves, doctor.'

'That's OK. I'll meet regularly with you and your team to see how things are going and I'm available – and to you, Kate, if you like – to come and talk to you at any time. Maybe you can work with us over a number of sessions towards Arthur's full recovery.'

'That sounds great, doctor, don't you think, Arthur?'

'Great for you, Kate!'

'No, come on, Arthur. This is for us all. The girls will be so delighted to know that you're doing this for yourself.'

'Well, as you know, I said I was not that into the whole thing, but . . . I haven't done that badly trusting you so far, doctor.'

'You can trust me, Arthur. And you can trust all of your team.'

'I'll give it a go, a really good go. In for a penny, in for a pound, as my old granny used to say.'

'Do you know, Arthur, I really like your old granny. She is definitely a favourite of mine!'

'Yeah, doc, right.'

Thursday, 16 June 2016

Arthur returns a year later, looking fit and well. His mood is cheerful and his manner relaxed.

'Hello, Arthur. It's great to see you again. How have you been? You're looking fantastic.'

'As you can see I am a bit better than the first time we met, doctor.'

'Arthur, it's great to see you looking so well. And you really are well, aren't you?'

'Yes, I am certainly a lot better. A "New Arthur", I guess you could say.'

'Good, well I'm pleased to meet New Arthur. And tell me, what's made the difference for you, for the birth of New Arthur?'

'Where can I start . . . I'm very grateful to Irene and the team. CFT has been a fantastic experience. No cakewalk now, but, sure – look at me! I'm a different person.'

'Talk to me about that, Arthur.'

'I guess the first thing, doctor, was the shame and guilt. I was so full of those things all I could ever do was beat myself up. It's still a challenge, but I am much better at being *kinder* to myself.'

'How did that come about?'

'Irene's been great. And all the CFT group. I still find the talking difficult, but we stuck at it and over time we've been able to delve into my past, to understand why it made me feel the way it did.'

'Rather than just judging yourself by it?'

'Yes, and accepting more how I feel. I'm getting away from the mindset of thinking everyone's on the attack here, you know? I've learned that I can't fight all the time. You can't think clearly when your mind is a blur: all you feel is anxiety, all you can see are the dangers out there. Sometimes I can unwittingly bite the hand that feeds me. Do you know what I mean?'

'Yes, that seems perfectly understandable to me, Arthur. You have been trying to defend yourself all along by using such a critical voice.'

'But then Irene helped me imagine Granny's rice pudding. I had nearly lost that altogether!'

'Arthur, that image means a lot to you, doesn't it?'

'You bet! I had lost any image of kindness in my life. Even though it was all around me in Kate and with my girls, I was on the alert the whole time. It's no way to live.'

'Yes, it's both exhausting and destructive.'

'I am using mindfulness much more; we did it in the group

and, do you know, it's making more and more sense to me as I go on, too?'

'Yes, we are all on a learning curve here, Arthur. It's good.'

'Yeah, and in talking with Irene I'm seeing – and believing – that things were not my fault, at least not all my fault.'

'Things like?'

'Like my childhood. Look, don't get me wrong, I've got a fair bit to go on this, but I know now my childhood was not . . . my fault.'

'And you can see that more clearly now?'

'I always knew it. What's changed is now I really believe it, you know?'

'Do you remember, Arthur, when you told me that you felt you Lacked Moral Fibre – L.M.F.?'

'Oh, don't remind me. It's a bit embarrassing for me.'

'No, that's not why I bring it up.'

'Doctor, all my self-pity makes me cringe a bit now, thinking about it.'

'Arthur, it's not my intention to make you cringe. Quite the contrary.'

'Irene and the CFT group helped me realize that I was running on adrenalin 24/7, trying to go in two directions at the one time. It's not a good long-term plan, you know.'

'Yes, indeed.'

'It's amazing, really. Talk about not being able to see the wood for the trees. Jesus!'

'Arthur, how are Kate and your girls and all that?'

'They're great. You know, before I couldn't see any of my good fortune. I couldn't take myself away from my battles or appreciate my family and the good things we have. When Kate called it my endless catastrophic debate, that really struck a chord with me. She was spot on, as usual. Kate has a great way of cutting through the bull.'

'Yes, when I met Kate I was struck by how well you work together. You're a good team, Arthur.'

'Yeah, she's everything to me and the girls. But she's her own woman too.'

'She seems very patient and insightful.'

'Yes, she certainly put up with a lot from me!'

'So, tell me, Arthur, do you feel that your *battles*, as you called them, are over now?'

'Well, let's just say the peace talks are going on in my head, if you know what I mean?'

'And do you have other goals now?'

'Now I know I want to be more contented. I want some happiness and some peace.'

'And you feel these goals are achievable?'

'Yes, they are now.'

'This is something that you talked with Irene about?'

'Yeah, often. We've discussed how contentment is achievable.'

'How, Arthur?'

'Look, I love my family and my life. It's not too much to ask to be happy, with them, is it?'

'No, not too much at all.'

'I never want to threaten the peace in our home. They had been living in a jeopardy of my making. Weirdly enough, the atmosphere was a bit like the threats and the moods I grew up with.'

'Arthur, how do you see yourself now?'

'How do you mean?'

'I mean all the anger that existed. It is only one side of you, of course.'

'The truth is I am a gentle man. At least I hope so – or I am getting there. I'm certainly calmer now, that's for sure. What was it our politicians used to say? "A lot done. A lot more to do." Ha!'

'Yes, I remember that one all right. So, tell me, Arthur, can you feel more compassion for yourself now?'

'Ah, yeah, I do. It's all about being genuinely good to myself. I've learned that now. Look at me, I've already lost 20 kilos. And I'm doing the Ring of Kerry charity cycle in a few weeks. I mean, I'm no Stephen Roche, that's for sure, but I feel great just thinking about it.'

'So you're enjoying the cycling?'

'I love it. Kate and the two girls had a good laugh the day I put on my new Lycra gear. But I don't mind. Sure, all the auld fellas like me are wearing it nowadays.'

'Arthur, tell me more about the weight loss. There is more to your success, isn't there?'

'Well, the team in your Wellness and Recovery Centre really worked a good bit with me. It's a holistic approach. That's what you said. A healthy mind in a healthy body.'

'That's it, Arthur. There's no health without mental health.'

'I took a bit of convincing, but I chatted with my GP. She was keen for me to go too. Anyway, we decided to take a radical step with my diabetes and my weight.'

'You had gastric surgery, didn't you?'

'Yes, I did, and it's been amazing. I've had a gastric band put around my stomach and my weight is better. Look at me! And I am now entirely off insulin. Can you believe that?'

'Yes, I can. We never doubted you could do it.'

'To be honest, the procedure was challenging. And I still have to be careful what I eat. I get very full very quickly. I'm still getting used to that. But I'm proud of myself. I see it now: my weight was another kind of hostility to myself.'

'Now there is a load off your mind and a load off your body!'

'Yes, I like to think so. Irene says I have learned to look after myself. I'm no longer beating myself up like I used to. And, like you said, this is a holistic, "mindful" approach.'

'Yes, it is, Arthur – absolutely.'

'By the way, I'd like to say thank you. I appreciate that you didn't condemn me for some of my little rants and raves last year. I can be pretty obnoxious if I let my temper flare, I know. So thanks for that.'

'It happens. We don't believe in being critical of the critic!'

'Oh, and did I tell you that I'm back on the guitar?'

'Really?'

'It was a part of me that just disappeared with all the crap that was going on. I'd forgotten myself that I could ever really play guitar. I'm just doing a few numbers, country and western is my thing. I'd forgotten how great it is to make music. In saying that,

Kate and the kids don't always think it's so wonderful! I know she's happy I'm up and about. God knows, she spent enough time looking at me lying in bed all day.'

'So, Kate sees your progress?'

'Of course. She's so much a part of it. She has twisted my arm to go along to her mindfulness class.'

'And how are you finding that, Arthur?'

'Well, your team recommended that we both go, so I went to keep the peace!'

'Good. And I'm not bringing up old battles now, but have your issues with your old employer been resolved?'

'Would you believe it's still dragging on? It's nearly three years now. You know, I don't bother about it so much any more. I leave all that to my legals. My solicitor is all over it.'

'Could you see yourself ever going back?'

'Back to my old job?'

'Yes, your old job.'

'No, not there. That's very much in the past. But I have been looking around on the internet for something. Maybe something completely different. I have a few ideas. We'll see. Maybe I'll join your dream team full-time.'

'You never know, Arthur!'

'Sometimes, doctor, the thought that I will be punished for having my good times back crosses my mind. It's just fleeting, but . . .'

'That's Old Arthur talking, don't you think? That's not really how you feel most of the time.'

'That's true.'

'And as I said earlier, I'm very pleased to meet New Arthur. Along with your granny and her rice pudding!'

'Yeah, but not too much pudding, mind. I only imagine it now! Can't you see, doctor, now I'm watching my weight!'

'Absolutely! You're looking fantastic.'

'I am, amn't I? And I have learned how to take a compliment as well.'

Arthur's Journey

Arthur's is a story of a life saved by psychotherapy. Through the combination of CFT with good physical care he is now able to pursue a life better lived than ever before. His therapy allowed him to change his priorities and move towards a kinder, more loving, wiser self and this view of living, combined with better physical care, has been truly lifesaving for him and for his family.

Arthur's journey is also revealing because it tells us that finding wellness is never simple. His story tells us something real about the pursuit of the well-lived life. There is probably no one answer and no one person who can ever offer a definitive prescription for being well – and neither should there be. What is important is that Arthur says he has moved closer now to wellness than at any other time in his life.

Arthur's physical health improved and so too did his mental health. His gastric surgery led to the unloading of his excess weight and this is more than a practical marker of wellness. It is also a metaphor for his mental recovery. In this way, Arthur chose to unburden himself as much as possible of the stress in his daily life. Arthur is better able now to free his mind for living in the present and he is more mindful than at any other time in his life. His CFT has been a mindful response to his many difficulties. Now he practises mindfulness and, perhaps even more importantly, he lives in a mindful way – really present, more kind to himself and others, and far less judgementally.

It is important to understand that Arthur's anger and his protest were not in themselves the source of his problem. Anger and protest can also be very positive emotions. As human beings, it may be right that we are angry and sometimes it is essential that we protest, especially when we are confronted by injustice. It may be that Arthur was right to confront his bullies and try to press on his superiors his views regarding the state of Ireland's economic affairs. His views were at least as valid as others offered at that time, but Arthur's anger and protest were not his only problems.

So what then made Arthur depressed and suicidal? It would be easy to suggest that Arthur had a biological illness arising naturally in the setting of a strong family history of depressive illness. It could be said that, under the pressure of the many stresses he was experiencing, Arthur's inherited tendency to depression was bound to emerge. Arthur very nearly succumbed to all of this, but an inherited tendency seems too easy an explanation for me.

Arthur's response to antidepressant medication had been unsatisfactory for some time. This points to a reality of therapy. Strategies that are not working need to be reviewed. Arthur's recovery emerged only when that medication was combined with CFT. It was this combined engagement with CFT and mindfulness that helped him recover. This combined approach was necessary to finally address his physical problems, his depressive issues, his shame and his self-reproach.

So long as Arthur lacked the ability to tolerate himself, he could not be expected to tolerate anyone else. His inability to soothe and calm himself stemmed from his early experiences and from the harshness of the world view he had been given as a child. 'It's a dog-eat-dog world,' he once said. In the end it was Arthur's shame and anger, his feeling of not measuring up to expectations that was actually eating him up. He had been so critical of himself that he felt like an outsider. This depression very nearly destroyed everything good in his life.

The behavioural tools he learned in CFT have stood to him. He has learned to tolerate distress and to accept his emotions. He has also learned that his critical voice is an understandable defensive reaction to the harsh criticism he was taught to fear. Now he practises mindfulness and lives more mindfully in the present, with an ability to imagine warmth and to receive kindness that he never perceived before. CFT has enriched his life. Its agenda of kindness matched exactly his need for compassion.

What is more remarkable is that these self-soothing and compassionate skills can be learned by so many. These emotional attributes and skills can also be taught. The basic methods of BT and CBT can be amplified by this more compassionate agenda. We have already seen that therapy can help us to behave and to even think in more helpful and different ways. Further still, what Arthur has shown us is that CFT can help us to feel differently and so to engage meaningfully with an ever more compassionate agenda for a life well lived.

Patricia

PATRICIA IS A FORTY-FOUR-YEAR-OLD married woman. She asked her GP to make a referral for an assessment and treatment of her depression and her intermittent death wish. Her GP's letter explained the background. 'Patricia is new to my practice, so I don't have many details. She is a puzzle to me. I wonder whether she has a bipolar mood disorder or maybe something else. All I know is that she lived in Scotland for a number of years and during that time she attended a psychotherapist, but apparently to no avail. She denies many other mood-related symptoms but still tells me she is desperate for help. This is because she says her moods go up and down, sometimes with several dips in a single day.' Despite this, Patricia works for a bank in a very responsible position. Her husband and family are devoted to her, but she remains privately at odds with herself, intermittently despairing and suicidal.

Patricia's Initial Assessment

Every person in distress is different. Each individual has their own unique story to tell. Just how that story is told says a great deal about how someone has managed for years with their particular mental health difficulty.

Chronic stress or emotional pain is difficult for anyone to bear. Patricia is a very resourceful woman, but as we shall see her defence against this kind of pain had become a way of life. Part of her protective mechanism was to put plenty of emotional distance between herself and her history, to 'park it' somewhere and to lock it away in Pandora's box. At times of greater distress this was more

211

difficult to do. At these times Patricia felt as though she was observing her problems rather than participating in them, as though her life was unreal, as though everyone involved (including herself) was simply acting out the words of a play. This extreme of defence is known as 'de-personalization' and 'de-realization' and it is very common.

An imagined form of reality can be very frightening but it can also be comforting or protective to 'dissociate' in this way. A very simple example could be quite functional – the practice of keeping a diary. Private writing such as this enables our alter ego to consider reality and to experience a world that the public self finds intolerable. Even a childhood diary could do the same. No one knew that Patricia had such a diary and that the only way she would be able to share her story was to open it and reveal its painful content.

Patricia's referral letter was presented at our weekly meeting with the multidisciplinary team. We discussed a new therapy called Dialectical Behaviour Therapy (DBT) as a possible treatment. DBT is an adaptation of typical Cognitive Behavioural Therapy. Its philosophical concepts are derived from the German philosopher Hegel and its ideas of mindfulness are borrowed from Zen Buddhism. The therapy has since proved very effective for people with so-called emotionally unstable or 'borderline' personality problems and suicidal behaviours. It is in my view the greatest achievement of the modern era of cognitive behavioural psychotherapy. Professor Marsha M. Linehan, who developed the therapy, is a pioneer of effective mental healthcare. Although I have never met her, my reading of her work and my witness of the results of her therapy have left me with a particularly positive view. For me, she is a modern heroine.

Marsha Linehan's personal journey is very significant. At the age of eighteen, she was diagnosed with schizophrenia. She was subsequently given a full range of biological treatments, including major tranquillizers and even electroconvulsive therapy. None of these interventions met her needs or proved to be very effective in relieving her distress. She has since said that her problems were probably caused by an emotionally unstable personality. Later she became a mental health professional in her own right and found herself trying, yet failing, to help people with similar problems of emotional disregulation. She began by using traditional CBT but found that the therapy was not working.

Like other modern therapies, DBT emphasizes the value of recovery in the 'here and now'. The journey towards a life well lived prospers in a compassionate therapeutic alliance rich in objective validation and empathy for those in emotional distress. DBT promotes ideas of mindfulness, acceptance and compassion, as well as structured learning using behavioural and cognitive methods, just like other therapies discussed in earlier passages of this book. It delivers these in a familiar behavioural and psycho-educational matrix, teaching skills, making diaries and using real-life exposure, but in DBT the therapy is enhanced by specific concepts, with focused groups, and telephone and media support.

So, what makes DBT so special?

Dialectical Behaviour Therapy (DBT)

DBT is different from other forms of therapy. It sees the problems of emotional regulation in a more holistic and connected fashion. In DBT, as in life, everything is in flux. Reality is full of opposing forces. Nothing is absolute. In this therapeutic mechanism the validity of each person's point of view is respected. Rather than defending the value of any one position or seeking to 'correct' the other, a DBT therapist recognizes the opposing, or so-called 'dialectical', stance. The discovery of a well-lived life is aided by skills learned in DBT and this education begins with the valid-ation of each person's experience and perspective. As Linehan puts it, 'Instead of looking for the validity of a person's behaviour in the understanding of their past, [we find] this validity in the current moment.' Traditional ideas of empathy in other forms of therapy are rooted in an understanding of the past, but DBT moves towards a recognition of the validity of each person's ideas in the 'here and now'.

In practice, DBT goes further, proposing that individuals in distress have an inherent wisdom about their experience, a so-called 'wise mind', even if this wisdom is not immediately apparent. This is a belief in the potential of every human being. It assumes that each individual is capable of wisdom with respect to his or her own life. As Linehan puts it, 'The DBT therapist trusts the patient has within herself or himself all that is necessary for effective change. The essential elements necessary for recovery are all there in the current situation.' Linehan sums up this humane confidence beautifully by saying simply, 'The acorn is the tree.'

We have already seen the value of mindfulness in other modern therapies. Arthur's successful experience of Compassion Focused Therapy (CFT) is a good example. The individual validation offered in DBT is the beginning of a similar journey through mindfulness, radical acceptance and self-compassion, but there is a crucial difference. While DBT acknowledges emotional distress, it seeks to reconcile it with the need to limit the damage done by persistent emotional inflammation. This is the essential paradox or 'dialectic' in DBT: living life well involves acknowledging the need for acceptance and at the same time the need for change.

'Dialectical' thinking is the skill of arriving at the truth through an exchange of logical arguments. This form of thinking acknowledges contradictions and so DBT appreciates the tensions that exist between apparently opposing positions. Actually DBT values these apparent contradictions. It holds on to them and seeks to balance them. As we shall see, this is a mindful approach. A right way of thinking, a set of absolute truths, is never defined or finalized. Thus DBT is a challenge to previously accepted CBT wisdom. The pursuit of recovery in DBT, the pursuit of the life well lived, comes through the therapist and the patient learning to experience reality in an entirely different, more balanced way.

To illustrate this, Marsha Linehan encourages us to imagine the DBT therapist and the man or woman in therapy as individuals sitting on opposite ends of a see-saw. The progress of DBT involves a constant movement of ideas and behaviours oscillating between the opposing ends of this dramatically poised scale. The dialogue

of recovery in DBT moves back and forth as though this relationship were a pendulum. As DBT skills are learned over time, the
individual and the therapist move closer towards a new, changed
and less turbulent equilibrium.

Some of us are more sensitive or more impulsive from the
very start. Each of us is unique. Biological, psychological, social
differences exist between all of us. According to DBT the origin of
emotional disregulation lies in two common sources: the
biological and the environmental. On the one hand, biological
factors (genetic or developmental) predispose each person to his
or her distress. On the other hand, the environment significantly
impacts upon us in unforeseen ways. Ultimately these two vectors
– biological and social – interact with each other either construct-
ively or destructively. Over time these inputs can lead to the
growth of a characteristic set of emotional problems.

Emotional instability is not a pejorative term. It refers to a
pattern of human behaviour associated with recurring self-
destructive acts, suicidal feelings and behaviours. When these are
experienced repeatedly, a very real pattern of emotional and
behavioural difficulties arises. And all this tends to happen again
and again and again. Many people struggle for years in this way,
as if propelled on a rollercoaster, their emotions rising and falling,
trying all the while unsuccessfully to resolve contradictory feelings and points of view. Such conflicts are characteristic. They
may be expressed in contemporaneous statements like 'I want to
live' and yet 'I want to die'. Emotional instability explains why some
people seem to seek help and yet reject that help at the same time.

DBT therapy is not an obscure practice. As we shall see its
behavioural methods are very practical. It teaches living skills and
it is focused on everyday life. DBT therapy works best when it
engages the patient, the therapist and the whole team, whether in
one-to-one sessions, in groups or by telephone and social media
support. Many adaptations of this therapy exist, but essentially
DBT is always about helping people who experience emotional
difficulty to reconcile opposing forces within themselves. The
benefits are measurable and they are very hopeful. The results of

DBT have established it as a new and positive route to a life well lived.

The Practical Skills of DBT

My favourite DBT resource is the *Dialectical Behaviour Therapy Skills Workbook*.[1] It's helpful to encourage people to use a workbook as they progress through the therapy, as their journey needs to be accessible and clear. The workbook is a collection of practical DBT exercises promoting the four DBT skills, which are:

- Distress tolerance
- Mindfulness
- Emotional regulation
- Interpersonal effectiveness

With a DBT workbook, recovery becomes more structured and easier to measure and maintain, but no book is a substitute for DBT delivered as part of an agreed therapeutic care plan. Each DBT skill has a basic and advanced level and each level may be progressed in learned steps clearly annotated by a behavioural diary of charts, feedback and real-life exercises.

All this may sound very intense, and even a little off-putting, but the effect is actually the reverse. Individuals in DBT find the transparency and clarity of its approach one of its most validating elements. It speaks to another common aspect of all effective modern therapy: it is egalitarian. After all, we are all in this together. Life is hard. We all experience its distress at some stage and so we all need methods to get us through. Some of these strategies may be more helpful than others. DBT proceeds with exercises to promote the recognition of self-destructive coping strategies such as worry and anxiety, avoidance and anger, and alcohol or substance abuse. Other common self-destructive

---

[1] McKay, Wood and Brantley, *The Dialectical Behaviour Therapy Skills Workbook*, New Harbinger, 2007.

coping strategies include self-injury, over- or undereating, sexual risk-taking, suicidal behaviours and despair. In DBT the individual learns to use alternative strategies aimed at promoting more functional tolerance of distress. These include methods for distraction and self-soothing. Changing attitudes is essential. The aim is to arrive at a radical new acceptance of the self. This is a concept we have already witnessed. In the case of Laura, she recovered using Acceptance and Commitment Therapy (ACT).

Distress tolerance includes distraction, but this is not the same as avoidance. Alternative actions can be seen as skills and they are best maintained when they are pleasurable and rewarding. It is necessary to be able to distract ourselves. We can do this in many ways: by paying attention to something or someone else, by engaging in alternative tasks, by developing an alternative set of thoughts to care about and enjoy. These may be as simple as counting things like our breath, the seven-times table or even sheep! The bottom line is that DBT encourages each person to develop their own personal distraction plan, to write it down and then to do it.

Distress tolerance also means learning ways to relax and soothe ourselves. DBT teaches people to reconnect with all the senses: smell, sight, hearing, taste and even touch. Someone in DBT might be encouraged to visit somewhere with a pleasant smell, like a bakery or a coffee shop, or to find a picturesque sight that is soothing to view, it might be they are encouraged to listen to music that brings them calm, or to savour the taste of a favourite food, or even just to play with a pet dog. These soothing actions could actually be on someone's list. Any of these actions could potentially give someone an experience of gentleness and kindness. In DBT each person is encouraged to develop their own distress tolerance plan using all five senses, to write it down and then to put it into effective action.

DBT teaches very practical and personal methods of distress tolerance to people at times of great distress. Distraction and self-soothing can be learned and so can mindfulness. This is key to DBT. It's helpful to take time out and to live mindfully in the present moment. Mindfulness techniques are not clichés. DBT promotes mindfulness as a key wellness skill. This involves the practice of meditation and exercises that teach us to imagine ourselves in more peaceful, serene settings.

One of the less obvious features of modern therapy is the way in which it promotes the imagination as a restorative human faculty in mindfulness. We may lose our imagination in the darkness of emotional pain, but a restored imagination can lead us out of this nightmare. Imagination can sustain us and restore our vision of a life well lived. Imagination is a far more powerful cognitive faculty than 'realists' would have us believe.

So each person in DBT is encouraged to develop a set of alternative coping strategies and to practise these daily in real life. Mindfulness is taught in DBT exactly as it is within CFT and ACT, and all of these techniques are enhanced by the ability to use the imagination, so as to transport oneself to a more peaceful time, to a calmer place and hopefully to a more complete sense of wellness.

Mindfulness in DBT can be remembered more easily by using the acronym 'FLAME'; where 'F' is for focus, 'L' is for letting go, 'A' is for radical acceptance, 'M' is for a 'wise-mind' and 'E' is for effectiveness. This 'E' is the ability to genuinely accomplish new goals. In these ways DBT helps each person to tolerate distress and to explore mindfulness further, to turn away from their emotional turmoil towards stillness, silence and peace.

DBT also teaches other skills to improve emotional regulation and to improve interpersonal effectiveness. To understand these aspects of Dialectical Behaviour Therapy perhaps we need to see how it works in real life. So now let me introduce you to Patricia. Let us witness her DBT journey to a life well lived.

Patricia's Journey Begins

Tuesday, 7 July 2015

At our first meeting Patricia is wearing a dark tailored suit and carries a large handbag. Above the brim of her bag is perched a small laptop computer and a number of well-worn notebooks.

Patricia's manner is immediately forceful, determined and impatient. She speaks first without any hesitation.

'I have come straight from work! What a dash in the rain! If you don't mind, I'd rather not waste much time with all the preliminaries. Can we cut to the chase?'

'Sure, Patricia, but your GP tells me he doesn't have much background from you. Is it OK with you if I ask you for some details?'

'Look, I spent two years on a psychiatrist's couch in Edinburgh. Bawling my eyes out, once a month. Just bawling and bawling. Talking treatment! It wasn't for me. Didn't even get to tell him half the stuff I had inside me. It didn't work for me. This time I'm ready to do things differently. So the question this time is, will you or your people help me?'

'I hope so, Patricia. We're here to help you.'

'I am convinced there is something "chemically" wrong with me. The older I get, the clearer that is becoming to me.'

'Mental distress can have many causes. It's rarely down to one thing alone.'

'Maybe, but I am here for a bit of the "magic". I need some relief. At this stage I want a medication that will stop the demons in my head.'

'Medication?'

'Yeah, you're a doctor, aren't you? There have to be some good drugs that you know about.'

'Why don't we talk first?'

'I thought you'd say that, but I explained to you that I am all out of *talk*. And I am all out of tears as well. Not that my emotions are drained completely. They are like a yo-yo; they go up and down, sometimes several times in a single day. I can't afford to let you go anywhere near them! Let's do away with the talk.'

'How can we make progress if we don't talk?'

'There may be another way. Can you see, I brought this notebook with me?'

'What is it, Patricia?'

'This, Jim, is my childhood diary – well, one of them.'

'Right, I see. Tell me, what age were you when you wrote this?'

'This one? About fourteen.'

'Can you tell me what you were like at that age?'

'Picture me. I was a tall, skinny, tomboyish, typical teenager.'

'And you kept a diary every day?'

'That's right, and now I am going to read some of it to you.'

'OK, go on, that's OK.'

'If you want to understand the real me – whoever that is – it's probably best starting here. You see, I've been reading this one over and over, as I do regularly, and there's something you have got to understand. This person – it's just not me any more.'

'It's not you?'

'No, I can't describe it. When I read this, it's like an out-of-body feeling, another person, you know?'

'Can you explain that to me, please, Patricia?'

'It's me, in so far as I wrote it – and it did happen. All this violence happened. Really. But I have no feelings for the girl in that situation. It's cut off. She's cut off. It's not that I have no sympathy – just no feelings, either way.'

'And how do you *feel* today, Patricia?'

'Today? Well, I suppose I feel like I've felt for years, for as long as I can remember.'

'And I take it that's *not* a good feeling?'

'No, Genius! It's definitely not a good feeling!'

'Maybe, Patricia, before you read your diary to me, if you wouldn't mind, maybe you would start by telling me how you feel today.'

'Perhaps, then, I will describe how I feel to you.'

'Do.'

'I will be brief. I feel like an iceberg on fire. I didn't just come up with that image recently. I've thought so much about it you wouldn't believe. I am in hell.'

'Hell? Patricia . . .'

'Yeah, real hell. And I want out. I want out of this hell, but I can't find my way.'

'But, Patricia, there must be a way, maybe it is just that it is not visible to us now.'

'That's why I'm here.'

'Patricia, can I ask you an important question: have you ever felt hopeless or even suicidal?'

'Sure, I have thought about it, and have even longed for it.'

'What stops you from acting on that "longing"?'

'I suppose it's got to do with feeling the pain. I have felt the same level of pain, the exact same level of pain, for a long time now and there are no peaks, no troughs, no bipolar episodes. Just consistent hellish, joy-sapping mental pain.'

'So . . .'

'So I suppose to answer your real question, no, I am not suicidal. It's like I came to a conclusion, somehow, I could take this pain, live with it. After all, I don't know how other people feel, really feel, inside. Maybe they're all the same as me. How would I know?'

'Does it have to be like this, Patricia?'

'Maybe, maybe not, but either way the pain is getting worse, or maybe I'm getting weaker, and I can't carry it any more. It's just got to stop. Sometimes I feel like someone is drilling into my skull. When I concentrate, it stops, but as soon as I turn away from work, the drilling starts again. This faceless, emotionless person, drilling into my brain.'

'What is there out there that helps you, Patricia? Anything that gives you relief, so to speak?'

'My pills, of course. And by the way, if you even suggest that I stop them, I'll be out that door quicker than *you* can say "I'm afraid our time is up."'

'No, no, Patricia, there is no suggestion of me doing that. If it's in your recovery plan, we are going to do whatever works, OK?'

'OK, good.'

'Is there anything else that helps you, Patricia?'

'Work. Work has saved me up to this point. I am in banking. I help people in financial trouble, sometimes desperate people buried in debt. I'm the friendly face of banking, or at least the more helpful side.'

'That sounds like an interesting job.'

'I love my work, and I'm very good at it.'

'Why wouldn't you be, Patricia?'

'That's a strange thing to say. I suppose because ordinarily my head is so full to bursting of distress that I can't get anything done. But my work takes my mind to a better place, a clearer place. I can function there, at work, pretty well.'

'That's good, I understand that, Patricia. So, tell me about your diary?'

'Yes, let's get back to that. Do you want to read it yourself, or would you prefer for me to read it?'

'Patricia, what would you prefer?'

'I think it's best if I read it, since it's written for me.'

'Go ahead then. I am listening.'

'I've picked out a couple of entries in particular. I'd like to start by reading them to you first.'

'Sure, like I said, I am listening, but don't worry if I make a few notes while you're reading to me.'

Patricia begins reading her diary calmly and without tears. She reads in a detached voice, as though she is retelling a story about someone else entirely. As we sit together in my room, listening to this account of a childhood of abuse and neglect, neither of us comments in any way. It is harrowing. It is as though a young Patricia has entered the room, in full voice, via these contemporaneous notes from her childhood. Patricia's past has been locked in her diaries and there it has remained throughout her adult life, secret, private, detached and apparently completely dissociated from her current being.

Tuesday, 21 July 2015

When Patricia returns, she greets me enthusiastically. Almost immediately she begins to read from her diary.

'I brought you another volume of my childhood chronicles! Can you bear to hear any more of them? I find reading to you is somehow new and different for me. It's cathartic, I suppose.'

'Are you happy to read some more?'

'Sure, actually I think it's essential. Now I have taken her out of my bag, I can't just put my younger self back in her place.'

'It's good to listen to her.'

'Can you listen to both of us?'

'Yes, let's listen together.'

'They started again this evening. It was pretty bad this time. We were in the middle of our dinner. Dad came home. I know he's not working so he must have been down in the Malt House, that horse-racing thing is on this week. I hate horseracing: little men whipping poor horses to go faster than the other little men. It should be banned. Dad seemed in good form at first, so we were worried, but hoping that they wouldn't start. He waved a bunch of tenners in my mother's face and said something 'bout Davy Lad (I think that's a racehorse). He was jeering at her, and she was just like stone, like he wasn't there at all. She knew that ignoring him drove him mad. She had poured loads of salt over his dinner, just as he was jeering at her. He didn't notice. I could tell it was going to start. The quiet before it starts is the worst feeling. Even the twins, who aren't even two years old, know that this is bad news. I knew I had to protect them. Last week a glass missed one of them by inches. At least the others know when to run and where. I dread it. I hate it. I hate them for putting us through this. Then Mam put his salty dinner down in front of him. He always sits at the head of the table, ignoring us, like we didn't exist. Not one of us looked up from our plates. I noticed Peter putting this hands up to his ears. I knew this was not good because he needs to know when to run. I gave him a little nudge under the table. There was some talk about "money" and "out of work" and "gambling" or something like that. And then he started to eat. My mother watched him, with a slight smirk. She didn't look or feel as terrified as the rest of us were. Then BANG! He flipped the dinner plate up with one hand and smashed it against the wall beside the stove. That was the signal, I shouted "RUN!" to the others, grabbed the twins under each arm and ran for the little cupboard under the stairs. I had cleared it out yesterday, so all of us could fit in there. I had also left a packet of fig rolls and a bottle of orange in

there, at the back, under the old boots, just for times like this. I tried to peek out, to see if there was any blood this time, but the noise of the shouting and smashing of plates made me close my eyes. The others just settled in behind me. No crying: they know that's not the thing to do when this happens, that makes things worse, much worse. My mother was swinging her bread knife wildly, really swinging it and swearing, shouting, "You f***ing lazy bastard!" My father used his favourite, the C-word, for her, over and over. I hate swearing. If I ever have a family, I will never swear in front of my children. Never ever. I heard one of the boys using the C-word the other day. He doesn't know what it means. I don't really know what it means. Then my father saw me peeking out through the cracked door. He stopped. My mother stopped too. They looked at each other. He made a run for the stairs. I nearly peed I was so frightened by him, by them. Then he just slammed the door and shut the dead bolt and that was it. Darkness. The fighting stopped after a while and the kitchen went quiet. I don't know where they go after these rows. Just as well I had the bottle of orange in there. I could smell the twins' dirty nappies, and the boys were starting to sob. After about an hour (but it felt to me like a lot more) the dead bolt suddenly opened. I gave it a good twenty seconds, then I pushed the door open, just slightly. Once the coast was clear, I led them all out into the kitchen. Smashed plates and food all over the floor. I whispered to the boys to go straight to bed, which they did, and I changed the twins' nappies, put them to bed and started cleaning up the mess again. I don't know where my parents went. I don't know what they do after these rows. At least they're not here. At least it's over. It's over until the next time. Soon as I'm old enough I'm gone anyway. As far as I can go. I hate my life here.'

Patricia lifts her head slightly and places her diary gently on her lap. Tears are coming down her cheeks. She takes some tissues from my desk and wipes her face.

'I am sorry to share this with you. It's an appalling account.'
    'Just hearing it is heartbreaking.'

'I feel like I am back there "under the stairs".'

'Like you were then, with the twins.'

'In reality, me and my childhood self, we're completely cut off from each other. I have left that person and moved on!'

'Maybe so, but imagine if you could be together or at least in better balance . . . that might be the way to go.'

'Imagine that!'

Tuesday, 4 August 2015

Patricia returns for another session. This time her manner is calmer.

'Hello, Patricia, it's good to see you.'

'Thanks for seeing me so soon again, Jim.'

'That's no problem. I am always happy to see you.'

'That's good to know, Jim. Somehow I feel like I am just starting out. I am not sure I have the courage to go through this.'

'You have, and it's good to start afresh. Let me begin with what might seem like an odd question: Why have you come here *now*? Of course you are here for help, but what made you do it now? Why *now*, Patricia?'

'Look, Jim, you're not the first psychiatrist I've seen, if that's what you're getting at. I have tried to find my Dr Feel-Good many other times.'

'Yes, you've told me of the years of weeping in Scotland. Has nothing really worked for you before?'

'No, like I said, I have seen a few other "gurus" before.'

'Well, there may be a very good reason for that, Patricia.'

'What's that?'

'Real solutions, Patricia, don't come from "gurus". They come from within yourself. Getting well is not about finding a Dr Feel-Good. You already have everything you need to succeed.'

'I have to say, Jim, that sounds a bit pop psychology to me. I didn't come here for you to read me some guff about the power of positive thinking. I can get that from the magazines out there in your waiting room.'

'That's fair enough, Patricia, but go on then, tell me – why did you come here and why now?'

'Well, I want some solutions to my life. I need answers. Why are my moods so difficult? Why is it so difficult for me to get on with everyone else? The only thing I can do well is work. I want to live well. I have kept my marriage and family going, but only just. I have been very successful in my career, but I am tired of being a – a dragon!'

'Are other people in your life telling you that things have to change?'

'Yes. Everybody. They all say they have to walk on eggshells around me. I can't see it, but I feel frustrated too because I should be better than this. I should be capable of so many things. I should be doing so much. But instead all I feel is ashamed and guilty – or bored and frustrated, and I don't understand.'

'One thing I can help you with is this word "should". Let's just say we don't do it around here. Let's try not to do any more of "should" – no more "should" do this or "should" feel that. Not here. Let's try and make this room a "should-free" zone.'

'That sounds like a recipe for anarchy to me! I'm not sure I follow you completely but, if you say so, whatever it takes. I told you last time all I want is to be out of my hell.'

'Yes, that's what's most important. That's also partly why your diary is so important.'

'It's strange, but I am always so certain in my diary. It's like my diary is another person entirely.'

'Maybe that is because your feelings are always *valid* in your diary. You can translate your distress into words in your diary and nothing is lost in translation. In your diary your emotions and experiences are respected and understood.'

'I never thought about my diary that way. There has not been too much respect or understanding of my feelings in my life so far. Maybe Little Patricia in the diary copes better than I give her credit for.'

'Maybe so. I see you brought your diary with you again today.'

'Yes, I thought maybe I'd need it to read some more for you, if you wanted?'

'Yes, but let's first talk, Patricia, about what you read to me last time. Can we?'

'OK. Oh – but before it goes out of my head, I was thinking about your question last time. You asked me, was there anything that helps me? Gives me relief from my hell? Do you remember?'

'Yes, Patricia, I do. Basically you told me that your pills helped and that your work was a distraction, isn't that right?'

'Yes, but there was one more thing.'

'Something else that gives you relief?'

'Yes. Something I haven't told you about yet.'

'And what's that?'

'I burn myself.'

'I see. And how does that help?'

'It gives me relief. It's difficult to explain to someone, so I don't talk about it. I've been doing it for years. I'm not sure why it started. I didn't put it in my diaries. Maybe I was afraid someone would find out and try to stop me from doing it. I need to do it. I've been doing it since my teens.'

'And what about the pain, Patricia?'

'What about the pain? What about the relief more like! The relief from my real pain! What about that pain?'

Patricia sits for a moment. Her agitation gives way to a sense of resignation as she speaks about things in her life she is used to keeping hidden.

'You know, Jim, I cut myself sometimes too. But I mostly burn. Burns are a lot easier to conceal, you know? Clothes and make-up and the likes. Cutting can be messy. I'm sure you know that.'

'Is anyone aware of this, Patricia?'

'No. Just me and my husband – and now you, of course.'

'Patricia, do you want to try and stop this self-harm?'

'Self-harm isn't my problem. I see my self-harm as a consequence, not a cause, of my difficulties. But I expect you will see it differently. Ending it could be part of my healing, but that's for another day, don't you think? It's no big deal – well, not for me anyway. I just wanted you to know. The whole story. But it's no big deal.'

'Patricia, most people think this is a big deal, but it's interesting that you don't.'

'Well, when you've been doing it for as long as I have, you know, it's kind of par for the course, as they say.'

'I see, Patricia.'

'No, you don't see, Jim – that's the point. I hide all my scars.'

'And that helps?'

'For a time, anyway.'

'Could we maybe talk about something else, Patricia? Going back to your parents, your childhood? I'd like to know a little more about who you are.'

'Sure, we could talk about that stuff all day long, but I want some effective action for how I feel. There's lots to say, as I'm sure you could tell from what I read for you from my diary.'

'How do you see your childhood experiences, Patricia? Do you see them as abusive? Would you say you were physically or sexually or emotionally abused as a child?'

'I suppose it's hard to define "physical abuse", isn't it? I mean judging by today's standards, everything's different.'

'No, I mean the type of violence that your parents traded with each other, did that ever actually come your way?'

'For sure, you got a slap if you were "bold" or "acted up" out in public. You know, at Mass or some event like that, where the neighbours could see. But it was no more than any of the kids I knew growing up would get. It was nothing like what my parents did to each other.'

'What about sexual abuse?'

'No, I don't think so . . . Actually, I can't say for sure. All I can say is that I don't recall anything like that.'

'And emotional abuse, Patricia?'

'That's different. Of course. I remember plenty of that. Plenty. "Emotional abuse". Yes, that definitely describes it.'

'Can you talk to me some more about what that was like? I am sure it's all there in your diary.'

'Not everything is in the diary. I wish it was. It would be better there. Unfortunately, too much of it's still in my head.'

'And perhaps in your heart, Patricia?'

'Of course, but even though I was a child writing it, I didn't understand it. Now, looking back, I can see that my childhood was chaotic. It was never safe. Their drinking and their violence added to the fact that my father was not bringing in much money. There was no one looking after me, or any of us.'

'You were the eldest?'

'Yes, so I would come home and try to get the dinner on and see there was something there for the younger ones. I helped them with everything, their homework, dressing, you name it.'

'No one thought that *your* needs were important?'

'My mother was tougher than my father in that way. As far as she was concerned, we were just meant to drag ourselves up and make no fuss.'

'And you said that your father wasn't working?'

'Yes, he had been laid off, as they say. I found out in school shortly after that "laid off" actually meant that he'd got the sack – he had struck a work colleague. The guy he hit had a son in my class and he let me – and the rest of the school – know exactly what really happened.'

'That could not have been easy on you, in school, Patricia.'

'No, the other kids would snigger and act like they were drunk, fighting, in front of me.'

'Children can be cruel, Patricia.'

'Yeah, I suppose, it didn't bother me much then. I got the real deal at home, so kids in a playground was . . . well, I'd take that any day.'

'And where had your father worked?'

'In a solicitor's office in the town.'

'And he was violent in work?'

'Well, one day anyway. He came back after a liquid lunch, got in an argument with his boss and clocked him. The guy was out cold seemingly. So the other kids told me anyway.'

'And your father was sacked?'

'Are you surprised?'

'No, not at all. And this led to some tension between him and your mother?'

'There was tension there before that, as long as I can remember. But when the pay cheques stopped, let's just say Mother was not best pleased.'

'That really put extra pressure on the marriage?'

'Yes, it did. I offered to get a job, you know, like the good kid. I said I'd leave school and get a job to help out.'

'And did you?'

'No, my mother laughed in my face. Said nothing, just laughed in my face. But my intentions were good.'

'I'm sure they were, Patricia. And have you ever tried to talk to them about what was going on in the house or about how you felt?'

'I would be afraid of what I might do to them. I did try with my mother long ago, but she just dismissed me. Said I was exaggerating. Told me the other ones didn't do any complaining, so why should I?'

'She blamed you?'

'Yes, I suppose so. She said I was always too sensitive. So, yeah . . . she dismissed me. Said I was just a whinger. She used to say that even as a baby I was a whinger. I'm sure I wasn't.'

'I am sure of that too!'

'How was I to know? I suppose I was sensitive back then, but I was only a teenager. She said I had to pull myself together.'

'And what did you think about that?'

'I just knew I was desperately unhappy and I suppose I blamed myself for that. As far as I was concerned, I couldn't get out soon enough. First chance I got.'

'Tell me, Patricia, do you take after either your mother or your father? Which one of your parents are you most like?'

'My father. Definitely my father. Even with all that went on, I admired his work. I loved the idea of working, earning your own money, doing something you liked.'

'You wanted to work in the law, like your father?'

'No. A journalist. That was my childhood dream profession. I think that's why I kept a diary. I think I believed I was like one of those journalists reporting from a war zone, you know, like John Simpson of the BBC.'

'And your diary helped you to get by?'

'Oh, yes, it did. It's like I was there, in the middle of it, with all the bombs and violence and horror, and I was just reporting on it, you know? In my imagination I wasn't the real target. I'd get to go back to a normal life when it was all over.'

'Well, in a way, Patricia, that was very true.'

'Yes, but my parents' moods and fights never stopped for long. When I got older, I always dreamt of confronting them. Their attitude was always so black and white, so simplistic. They always blamed me by saying that if I just worked harder at school and didn't take things to heart and didn't complain so much that things would be so much better for everyone.'

'Do you feel there was any truth in their analysis?'

'Of course. I wished at times I was more robust. As you might say, more *resilient*. I suppose I never knew who to trust or how to control my feelings in a normal way.'

'Do you feel you know that now?'

'It can't be normal to feel this unhappy or this hellish. This up and down all the time.'

'Would you like to have a more emotionally stable life, a life better lived?'

'Wow, that would be good. Have you got one on the menu?'

'I could check with the kitchen!'

'Ha ha! Jim, I wish it was that easy. Do you think I'm crazy, Jim?'

'No, not at all. I think you are very distressed and I'm sure that you can be better.'

'How?'

'If we looked at things differently, if we worked together, without blame.'

'Sounds reasonable, go on.'

'Have you ever heard of a therapy called DBT, Dialectical Behaviour Therapy, Patricia?'

'I've heard of CBT. The guy in Scotland talked lots about it.'

'Well, DBT is a development of CBT but different. I think it might help to move you towards that better place, if you were willing to try it?'

'What makes you think it will be any different this time?'

'DBT is a new approach with lots of evidence behind it. You could make a start by meeting with my team, on a weekly basis, maybe in groups and with me, if that suits?'

'Look, Jim, I don't want you to pass me off to any old therapist after a couple of sessions and then have me just check in every year.'

'No, Patricia, that's not the way we do things. I have no intention of palming you off to anyone. I would be very much part of your team. We are all in this together.'

'Are we? Well good, then. Because I feel there is still a lot more of me and my diary that I need to talk about.'

'That's fine with me, Patricia. Maybe for our next meeting bring along your diary, if you like?'

'Now I take it everywhere with me. It's like a lucky charm, or maybe the opposite.'

'Maybe it's both at the same time?'

'Maybe.'

'And will you think about the DBT as well? I have some litera-ture on the basics of it, if you're interested?'

'Can you email that to me, please? I wouldn't want to let that fall out of my handbag at work.'

'Consider it done, Patricia.'

Tuesday, 18 August 2015

Patricia is finding it difficult to speak out loud about feelings she has kept hidden for so many years. There is a sense of impatience but also fear at letting go.

'Difficult, Patricia? How do you mean?'

'Well, I found our last session extremely difficult. It was for me, at least.'

'I am sorry, I hadn't realized that, Patricia. But each time we meet, we do talk about some very painful things. These are things that are difficult for anyone to talk about.'

'Well, it wasn't what we talked about – more how we talked about it.'

'Sorry, Patricia, did I say something to offend or upset you?'

'Well, actually yes, you did. A few things, they've been spinning around my head for the last couple of weeks since.'

'Oh, Patricia, it's not my intention to hurt you.'

'It was more your attitude – at times, your silly jokes, your behaviour really did hurt me. I just got the impression that you don't like me, and if you don't like me, how can you really help me?'

'Well, I can tell you straight up, Patricia, that I don't dislike you and I don't do impressions.'

'This is what I mean, that kind of reply. What are you doing making silly jokes? I'm here baring my soul and you're making smart-arse comments.'

'Sorry, that's not my intention, Patricia, not at all. Please forgive my attempts at humour.'

'Well, I just think that you don't realize how hard it is for me to come here, going through all this and then going out and facing all the things in my life as though nothing had been said.'

'What are you facing now?'

'My painful life! My responsibilities! Outside of work, I can't get anything done, I feel like such a waste of space sometimes, and so bored, I really do.'

'Patricia, have you ever thought about how brave you are?'

'Me? Brave? No, not for a long time. At a couple of points in my life maybe, but not now.'

'Well, it seems to me that in many ways you have been heroic.'

'Ah, come on now, Jim. You see, this is what I'm talking about: one minute you're saying to me, maybe my parents had a point about me whining and whinging all the time, and the next you're telling me I'm a superhero! Gimme a break, doc, will you? It seems to me that if you're not having a go at me, you're patronizing me.'

'I am not having a go or patronizing you in any way, Patricia. Really, I'm not.'

'Well, that's how it seems to me, Jim.'

'Look, Patricia, when I said to you that I don't do *impressions*, I meant it. I wasn't being a smart-arse, not at all.'

'What – what does that even mean, though? What do you mean by not doing impressions? Tell me!'

'I mean that we are both being "real" here. I am here for you. My team is here for you. Is there any harm in that?'

'There could be. For one thing, you could all be wasting your bloody time.'

'Patricia, I'm certain that this need not be a waste of anyone's time.'

'Well, you may be certain, but I'm certainly not. What can an hour's chat with you really achieve? Sometimes with weeks in between. Let's not put a price on this here.'

'There is another way I could help you, Patricia, but it would involve more of your time.'

'Right, more time – and money, no doubt.'

'Patricia, did you have a chance to think about the DBT treatment I mentioned? If you remember, we discussed it at our previous session.'

'Yes, I did, and I had a look online about it too. Looks to me like there's a lot to take in.'

'Yes, there is lots out there about it, but we could take it in small chunks. It's a new avenue and there's a very good chance this will help you. A good place to start is with a DBT skills group.'

'What's a skills group?'

'Well, we have a DBT skills group here, we call it Living Through Distress.'

'Living Through Distress? Sounds about right to me.'

'Would you consider coming along, Patricia?'

'Maybe I will go, but just because I don't want another year to go by with no relief. I need to rid myself of this pain. I need the right help.'

'Well, this could be it, Patricia. Will you give this a go?'

'I want to. I really do. I guess that's your answer there, Jim, to the question you asked me at our earlier session too.'

'Remind me of that question, Patricia.'

'Why now? You asked me, "Why now?" Why am I here now?'

'And the answer?'

'This has to be *my time*. Now I need to be ready to take help. I'm all done fixing everybody else's problems. I am done hurting.'

'Patricia, do you know what a powerful realization you have come to? It's really something to say, "My time has come." To me that's heroic, Patricia.'

'Yeah, sure, enough with the Wonder Woman talk, Jim. I'm not there yet.'

'No, but maybe we are on our way.'

Tuesday, 1 September 2015

Patricia has started attending our DBT skills group. She has met with Clodagh, our DBT therapist, on several occasions now. She went to the group with no expectations and is surprised to have found it useful.

'Patricia, can we talk about the DBT skills group? What do you feel about Living Through Distress?'

'For one thing it's aptly named. There are a lot more people like me out there than most people imagine.'

'Fellowship can be good.'

'I suppose so. At least it means your therapist isn't wasting her time either. God, she works hard. I like her. What's her name?'

'Clodagh.'

'Yeah, that's right, Clodagh. She seems like she really cares. That's a good trick.'

'She does care, Patricia. You can trust Clodagh.'

'Do you trust her, Jim?'

'Yes, I know her work through Living Through Distress.'

'I suppose you do, Jim, but you can't know what it is like really . . . It's all academic to you, isn't it?'

'Not actually, Patricia. I am genuinely interested to hear how it's going for you. Could you tell me about it? Talk me through what it is you do there, tell me what you think is important.'

'Well, since you're asking, Clodagh's DBT training has four modules. The first one I found tough. It was all about learning to tolerate my distress. It was deep-end stuff, no messing about, but I think everyone appreciated that. After all it's not a bloody book club I joined!'

'Yes, indeed. But you got through it and you took some things from it. The team tell me that you really engaged from the start, Patricia.'

'There was no point in me going if I wasn't going to engage. Besides, the team is great. No judgement – that's not for me. I need action.'

'Good.'

'Yeah, next up was the module on mindfulness.'

'Did you find that helpful, Patricia?'

'I really did. It's not the mindfulness I am used to. Like, I have bought books on it and I have a mindfulness app on my phone. But this was different.'

'Learning to tolerate distress and to be mindful. They are two great skills!'

'I am not there yet, Jim. There is an advanced level on all this and, anyway, putting all this into practice in real life isn't going to be easy.'

'For sure!'

'There are modules to come about regulating my emotions and managing relationships more effectively. That kind of stuff.'

'It's great you have engaged with it.'

'I found myself and Steven, that's my husband, having con-versations about my emotions in the evenings. Learning not to be so intense. Seemingly you can actually learn that too! Maybe I should have done this years ago.'

'But, Patricia, a lot of these learning methods are quite new, you know? They haven't been available for very long.'

'Well, I'm glad to be getting to know them now. I do feel I'm making real progress.'

'That's good. And some of the other modules, how were they?'

'I'm only starting the third one now, Emotional Regulation. It's going to be a challenge. So far I see it being kind of like anger management. I know that's not what it's called, but it is all about having more effective interpersonal relationships, reducing my chaos, not being as destructive when expressing my point of view. I will still express myself but hopefully in a calmer manner. This is a good development for everyone, I can assure you, Jim.'

'Of course. And there is the fourth module . . .'

'Yes. We haven't come to that one yet. It's more about being effective in the real world. I am getting there, but I'll take one skill at a time.'

'Tell me, Patricia, doing this must be such a challenge.'

'You know, Jim, it is a challenge, but it's different and I feel I am learning so much.'

'Tell me, are you still self-harming?'

'Yes, I still burn myself the odd time – but less frequently in recent months. Each time is a challenge, but I feel I have some new weaponry to deal with it now. New skills, I suppose.'

'So is that what you are taking from the skills group?'

'Yes, for sure. But let me tell you something quickly before we finish today. Steven booked us on a weekend away last week – a city break. We haven't been away in God knows how long. Anyway, it didn't start off too well.'

'Oh no, what happened?'

'I've always found airports unnerving places, especially now with all the extra security. I always feel like I'm being scrutinized, you know, accused of something suspicious.'

'Yes, well, the times we live in, Patricia.'

'Yeah, well, we had trouble at check-in: bags too heavy, they wanted another €20 or something. And I completely lost it with the guy. He was not being helpful at all. I told him that it was a scam that they had going and they were ripping people off who had no choice but to pay. So he called his supervisor and they made a scene. Well, OK, I was making a scene too, but their stuff was totally unnecessary.'

'And so did you pay the extra?'

'We had to! And they put us to the back of the line. I felt humiliated. Steven tried to cool me a bit before we got on the plane, which did work, for a while. And then this bunch of yobbos down the back of the plane started singing, you know? Yobbish behaviour. And I'm a nervous flyer at the best of times. So I asked the steward – calmly, mind – if she could ask them to stop.'

'And I take it that didn't work?'

'No. She pretty much ignored me and said nothing to these guys who were having a bar-room singsong at the back of the plane!'

'So?'

'So I asked her again, a little more forcefully this time, but she accused *me* of being the troublemaker and basically told me not to be a killjoy!'

'And how did you cope with the situation?'

'Steven tried to calm me, I took an extra pill and I sat there for the hour and a half or however long it was thinking about how as soon as I got to the hotel I was going to plug in my hair straighteners and, well, you know what.'

'Self-harm? And did you burn yourself?'

'No.'

'What stopped you?'

'No, idea, maybe it was Steve, maybe it was the DBT skills, some exercises I have learned. I tried to go to a better place in my head. I don't know which skills worked. Maybe all of them. But I didn't burn myself and that's all that matters to me at the moment. I feel I must be doing something right.'

'Yes, Patricia, you are. You can be proud of that, can't you?'

'Yeah, I felt good about it. We had a nice weekend. No more incidents. And I think I did Little Patricia proud.'

Tuesday, 15 September 2015

Patricia has been home to see her parents and describes her emotional response to the visit.

'You know, Jim, I decided I was going to go down home and confront my parents. Not in an angry way. It wasn't a spur of the moment decision; I allowed myself time to think about it. I even discussed it at Living Through Distress. Then I found myself on the M6, heading for home.'

'So what did you think prompted it exactly, Patricia?'

'Well, an anger rose in me – at you first, then later I realized it was them that I was really angry with, and I wanted to tell them to their faces.'

'And have you had much contact with your parents since you left home?'

'I am in contact with them intermittently. Family events, the usual, but no cosy chats, let's put it that way. That's not how we do things in our family.'

'And your siblings, do you see them much?'

'Some of them. I'm close to my sister Marian, or close enough. She's the newsfeed between me and the rest of them. She keeps me up to date. Sometimes whether I want to know or not.'

'But you are in contact with your parents, so to speak?'

'I don't know the last time I had an actual conversation with my mother, not since I was a girl maybe. She still rules with an iron fist over the rest of them – a real despot. I've known for a long time that I'll get no backing. When I'm talking about the past, they become very interested in looking at their shoes all of a sudden.'

'So you went to confront them. And what was it exactly that you were going to bring up with them?'

'Well, the violence, of course, the "emotional abuse", as you called it. The horrific atmosphere in the house. No child should have to live through that.'

'Wow! That was a big decision. How did it go?'

'It went exactly as expected. I went in, they were surprised to see me, but I got my usual warm welcome: "To what do we owe this pleasure?" my mother said sarcastically. I just got straight into it. I was calm, kept my voice low and I stuck to the facts. I was clutching one of my diaries, for support – from Little Patricia, you know.'

'Do you feel they heard what you were saying to them?'

'These people only hear what they want to hear. At first I got the usual "You need to get a grip on yourself" and "You're crazy – you're totally exaggerating what happened." But I persisted. I was surprised at myself how I didn't lose it completely with them. The level of denial we're dealing with here is astounding, you know?'

'So you said what you had gone to say. How did you feel?'

'Well, in the end they were just staring. Staring through me, like I was a ghost that they couldn't see – invisible. They were just standing there, staring. How did I feel? Maybe a little relief, but also, you know, I felt a bit of sorrow for them. Two old people, faced with their wrongs of the past, and denying I even existed, now or then, Little Patricia and me. Like I said, we're dealing with really serious levels of denial.'

'And so you left?'

'Yeah, I turned and left. Got in my car and headed home. I feel I handled my emotions well that day. I was actually very calm. It gave me a bit of hope for the future.'

'Lots of hope for the future.'

'Definitely!'

Tuesday, 13 October 2015

Patricia continues to work with Clodagh and the DBT skills group, Living Through Distress.

'You know, Jim, I want to tell you what happened to me at work the other day.'

'Of course, Patricia. Please go ahead.'

'Well, you know that I work in the finance industry, helping people out of debt. I told you that before, yeah?'

'Yes, you did.'

'Well, when I'm at work I'm really at work – 100 per cent, no distractions, no nonsense, total commitment.'

'You're very focused, Patricia.'

'I am. I have to be to deal with some really heartbreaking cases, families facing homelessness and the likes. I take my job very seriously. But obviously my clients don't need tea and sympathy: they need someone who can give them solutions, get them out of a mess, and that's me. I try to provide solutions. I don't involve my emotions. Don't let them get in my way, you understand?'

'Yes, yes I really do, Patricia.'

'So yesterday I had a typical enough case for the times we live in, unfortunately: a young family facing eviction. I've dealt with sadder cases, mind, but for some reason this particular case really got to me.'

'In what way, Patricia?'

'I just felt the tears and empathy rise in me like never before at work. So I had to promptly leave the meeting room and had a good cry in the Ladies. But it wasn't the visceral, painful crying like I normally have. It was different – like a sobbing for someone else's pain, empathic like. Not my pain – it seemed different. It seemed OK.'

'And you link this to your trip to see your parents?'

'Yes, I don't know why, but I do. And in a positive way. Maybe it's because they will never cry about someone else's pain. I don't want to be like that.'

'Learning about relationships, Patricia, is also part of DBT.'

'Do you know that Steven and I have been together for twenty-two years this summer?'

'And has your life together been happy?'

'Not always a bed of roses, Jim, but we get by. We're a decent team.'

'And your kids?'

'Yes, well not so much kids any more: adults now. Tom's twenty soon and Amanda's turning nineteen this year.'

'Talk to me about you and Steven.'

'What can I say about Steven? Well, he is the only person in the world that I actually trust. No one gets as close to me as him. Look, the kids are great, but they more . . . tolerate me, whereas Steven leaves me to myself when I'm having a meltdown. He can read me. He knows me.'

'A meltdown?'

'Yeah, you know . . . When I'm not working, I can be a complete nightmare.'

'Can you describe these times to me, Patricia?'

'I'm not sure if there are words to describe them. It's not just anger or frustration or even excitement – sometimes it's all of these things. I just can't get a handle on my emotions. Like I said, my emotions are all over the place and I go into meltdown mode.'

'What does Steven say about these times?'

'He thinks I'm manic. At times he could be right.'

'Does he ever think you have bipolar mood disorder, manic depression perhaps?'

'No, we went down that line with previous psychiatrists, but I am not bipolar: even when I am flying off the handle, I can always work and sleep. I have never done anything out of the ordinary. Or anything really off the wall.'

'You don't think you have ever been really high or manic?'

'No, but I do think that there is something wrong with my emotions. I'm very sensitive, so easily hurt, and these hurts – well, they just kind of grow and keep growing in my head. It's all so personal – they go straight to the heart.'

'How does that make you feel, Patricia?'

'Well, if something or someone upsets me with words or actions, I can't forget about it and just move on. I ruminate on it, go over and over it until it's the only noise in my head. There's no room for anything else.'

'But does this happen as much as before? Your life does seem better now. Better than before.'

'It's better. It's better now, OK, but that doesn't change how awful it was when I was a child and teenager. This is what's driving everything else in my head, I presume?'

'And so when you think about your emotional problems as a whole, what conclusions do you come to?'

'Look, my childhood was terrible, but that doesn't mean that I want a terrible adulthood, for things to stay as they are for the rest of my life.'

'That makes sense to me, Patricia.'

'The DBT group is really helping, I know that. We are learning how to manage our feelings. I have lots more I can do to soothe myself. I can have lots more pleasures . . . and not just guilty ones!'

'That sounds good.'

'I feel I am more able to calm my feelings, reduce that red mist so I can deal with relationships and emotions more clearly. I've always had trouble getting on with people, you know?'

'Why do you think that is, Patricia?'

'I suppose, maybe, I'm just not a very nice person.'

'Oh no, that's not how I see it.'

'Yes, of course you would say that. And that's what the DBT group say as well, but it's hard to change the experiences of a lifetime.'

'What about dealing with your self-harm?'

'It's reduced, for sure, but it hasn't gone away. When I get really desperate . . . But it's happening much less now.'

'So what do you do instead? How do you prevent it from happening?'

'This may seem crazy to you, but the other day I was frustrated at something or other, I don't even remember what, but I was getting that feeling I get before I burn myself. So I went upstairs to get the hair straighteners. And as I was plugging it in, waiting for it to heat up – you know, like you were waiting for a kettle to boil for a nice cup of tea – I started to laugh! I giggled at first, but then it was a good big belly laugh at the whole set-up. I know it sounds ridiculous. If anyone had seen me, God knows what they would think!'

'No, Patricia, not ridiculous at all. Laughing is much better than hurting.'

'Yes, anyway, I didn't burn myself that time. I pulled the plug out of the hair straighteners, went downstairs and put on the kettle and had that cup of tea, still laughing to myself. Weird, eh?'

'Maybe it's progress, Patricia. Were you at home alone when this happened?'

'Yes, I had popped back to the house for some lunch. I do that sometimes, you know, to take a break from the banal chitter-chatter of the workplace lunchtime, the noise. It really annoys me at times, you know? With all that's going on in this country, all these people want to talk about is celeb gossip. Christ, that's probably what had me riled in the first place.'

'You know, as part of your DBT treatment if you find yourself in a situation like that again, you can make a quick phone call. Someone can have a chat with you right then and there, and maybe just making the call will be enough for you to just take a minute, catch your breath, so to speak?'

'Yes, I understand that. We had a good discussion about that recently, and I have to say that it came as a big relief to the group – just to know that we wouldn't have to wait for weeks to talk to someone.'

'So you know we're there if you need us?'

'Yes, and I haven't felt the need yet, but it is a comfort to know – a bit like having your pills in your handbag. Just to know they're there.'

'On the topic of your medication, Patricia, how is that working for you?'

'I'm on the lowest dosage now. I have been for a long time – going back to when the kids were small, I'd say.'

'And how do you feel about that?'

'I feel good, of course. I know I warned you earlier to keep your hands off my pills, but the reality is that I don't want to be taking any more pills than I have to, especially if I don't have to. I don't think anyone really does, not for ever anyway. So I see myself as on the road to maybe some day no pills at all. Can you imagine that?'

'Yes, I can, absolutely. Getting back to Steven, if we may, Patricia?'

'Yes, Steven, he is my rock. I'd say that I would have drowned a long time ago only for him.'

'And do you see him as part of your recovery team?'

'Oh, yeah. He's even talking about coming along to one of our sessions maybe?'

'That would be fantastic, Patricia. I would like to meet him, as long as he and you are happy with it?'

'We'll see. It's just talk at the moment. I've been discussing the treatment with him a lot – what's been happening with the skills group – and he's interested, you know? He's never judged me, even when I've been a nightmare to live with.'

'And how has he coped with that, do you think?'

'He's practical and he loves me, I am sure. He's an engineer, so I think he likes to take a step back from a situation, try to calm it at first and then look for a solution. He has always supported me in my quest for professional help, always.'

'And the children?'

'What about the children?'

'How have they been over the years with your—'

'My meltdowns?'

'No, I didn't mean that. What I was asking was, what do you think their view is? From their position?'

'Yes, an interesting way to put it, Jim. I think that because of all the violence in my childhood there was never going to be any of that in our home. I was, and still am, determined to make sure that my children are not exposed to the horrors that I saw and heard. I've always been sure about this.'

'And Steven?'

'Of course we're united on that. He's a good shield for them. When the kids were small, I think I probably had my best years. I might go as far as to say that they were happy times. They were happy kids. We provided them with everything they needed, I'd say. I always knew that one day they'd fly the coop and for that reason I think I really concentrated on trying to enjoy their younger years. Steve did too.'

'And of course one day the children will eventually leave for good.'

'Well, they've gone already, Jim, as I see it. Once they leave for college, that's kind of it. Who knows where they will end up? It's a big world. I really want them to do what's best for themselves, I really do.'

'You say Steven was a shield for them. What do you mean by that?'

'In their teenage years, I felt I was going backwards. My outbursts, "meltdown moments", let's call them, were getting more frequent and more worrying. Steven was like the referee in a boxing match, you know? When one guy gets knocked down, he keeps the other guy away, at a safe distance, until he knows he's good to go on. Not that there was any boxing – we didn't do that in our house – but you get the idea.'

'Yes, I understand. It's not an easy role to play, trying to keep everyone happy.'

'No, but he did just that. He knew that there was something deeper. He didn't think that it would all come good by itself, but he has a way of acting in these scenarios. He's a "cool under pressure" type. It's kept us together – as a family, I mean. I'm sure of that.'

'It's good to be with someone like that, Patricia.'

'Like I said, he's my rock. You know, sometimes he reminds me of Little Patricia – that ability to be clear-minded in a crisis. I'd like to channel a bit of that myself. She was brave.'

'But you are brave, just like Little Patricia. She became you. You were never split except in your distress. You have all that ability that was in her . . . and more. You've proved it in the past.'

'Yes, maybe. I'm starting to see that . . . Have you noticed that I've stopped bringing my diary to our sessions?'

'I have noticed that, Patricia.'

'Yeah, I thought that we would read more entries as time went on. But that's not how it works, is it?'

'Well, it's down to you, Patricia. If you want to read more, then we could.'

'No, I'm not suggesting that. In fact, I'm happy to leave Little Patricia at home. I've stopped bringing her diary around with me in general. I still keep all my diaries in a safe place. I'll always want to keep them.'

'Maybe we only needed to read those pieces together. Maybe that was enough?'

'For now, Jim. I had never read it out to anybody before like that. I think it helped. It moved something, maybe.'

Patricia's Journey

Patricia continues to do well. She has maintained her association with our DBT therapy group, although she uses it less frequently. She recognizes that her childhood experiences were abusive, but she understands that her present and future need not be. She has discovered remarkable tools for resilience and a renewed determination to be well. She has found support in a therapy and so her recovery is continuing. Her DBT has been significant and it has helped her find the real remedies from within herself, remedies of distress tolerance and mindfulness, emotional regulation and effectiveness. DBT therapy helped her recovery to revive and grow again. Patricia has now recognized her need for acceptance of her past, whilst at the same time understanding the need for change in her present. As Linehan puts it, 'The acorn is the tree, and the tree is still growing.'

Thousands of words and hundreds of academic papers have been written about DBT and I will not attempt to rewrite them all here. Still, given the acknowledged benefits of this form of therapy, it is so surprising that more is not known about DBT in the wider community. This is, ultimately, one of the main reasons for writing this book: to make these real advances in mental health-care more widely known, more widely talked about and hopefully more widely available.

Still, for now it is worth considering why such progress in mental healthcare is not better known and why DBT is not in our consciousness in the way that CBT seems to be. For one reason, DBT has not been around as long as other forms of traditional CBTs. For another thing, its basis seems too complicated, too philosophical and its delivery too labour intensive. This is one reason for the many adaptations to DBT in mental health services in the community. These are a good thing.

That being said there is too little stomach for complexity in mental healthcare and so too little investment when it comes to complex solutions. When developments are made, the costs for these are invariably provided at the expense of some other much-needed programme. When we look for remedies, we still prefer quick fixes and cheaper, more didactic prescriptions. Rather than promote the value of mental healthcare we tell others publicly to value it *for themselves*. It's a pity. The truth is that mental healthcare is not something that we can restore for ourselves. And mental healthcare is not cheap. It is complex and human and challenging, and we will only make healthcare progress by acknowledging all of this.

The great news is that effective therapy is available in mental healthcare and DBT is one of the best examples of this offering. Rather than quote from the numerous papers, studies and reports (which are there for anyone to see), let me start and finish by declaring our own experience. It is fair to say that the introduction of DBT psychotherapy has been transformative of our mental health service. I have seen many clinical examples of this at an individual level, but for objective evidence of measurable progress across our service it is significant that levels of self-harm have fallen dramatically since our psychologists introduced DBT. They did this through our Living Through Distress skills group and since its introduction our outcomes reports have supported its effectiveness again and again.[2] In addition to a reduction in self-harm, it seems to me that general levels of therapeutic skill across our other multidisciplinary teams may have also risen and this is perhaps because of a greater awareness of DBT concepts in therapy. This increase in skill has been most apparent in our day-to-day management of conflict and dispute elsewhere, and across the whole of our mental healthcare service.

So the real question is this: how much do we care about people with emotional instability or other enduring personality prob-lems or mental health difficulties? Do we care enough to provide meaningful, effective therapy for these problems? It's not clear that enough of us do. If we really do care, then we will need to shift our focus away from our failed arguments, our harsh

---

[2] St Patrick's Mental Health Services (SPMHS) Outcomes Report, www.stpatricks.ie.

judgements, our dismissals and our pious homilies. We will need to recognize and accommodate mental health difficulties in some of the most troubled and enduringly distressed people in our community. Perhaps the economic argument alone will be compelling. Their high use of other health services and their excess morbidity and mortality are proof enough of the needs. Investment in effective treatment would be very good value by comparison to the alternative.

Joseph

JOSEPH IS A SEVENTY-FIVE-YEAR-OLD widower with Parkinson's disease. His GP wrote to me, explaining that Joseph's beloved wife of more than thirty-five years had died over a year earlier and since then he had not coped well. His only son was living in Italy and so Joseph felt completely alone. 'I fear he may have a severe depression and that he is actually longing for death,' the GP's letter said. 'I am concerned about his risk of suicide, although he denies this and says he is happy to see you. As he puts it, this may be his last chance of recovery.'

Joseph's Initial Assessment

Joseph had a long history of physical and mental illness treated elsewhere. His medical problems included raised blood pressure, raised cholesterol and also Parkinson's disease. While most of his care had been provided by his general practitioner in the community, his neurological diagnosis and treatment had been confirmed by a consultant neurologist.

We had never met before. With each initial assessment the perspective changes. My focus for Joseph was firmly on the present. My questions gently explored the background to each of his problems as they emerged. It was immediately apparent that Joseph's physical and mental health were intertwined. In time it would become clear that his psychological wellbeing was also inseparable from the whole of his health.

Joseph's face barely moved as he spoke at our first meeting. He sat forward in his chair, his pale hands trembled in his lap, as though he was rolling some invisible thread between the tips of his thumbs and his forefingers.

251

Joseph was able to tell me that he was depressed and that this had been his longest and most profound episode of clinical depression. His memory was not affected. According to Joseph, he had been depressed a number of times before but each episode had been treated successfully by former GPs. It seemed his previous episodes were of a similar character (although usually of shorter duration) but now, in Joseph's bereavement, his mood had not lifted with treatment in general practice.

This initial assessment would take time. There was a need to explore all factors in order to assist Joseph's recovery and to calmly gain his cooperation with all that was required to restore him to wellness. The care plan was not about one single therapy. Joseph's road back to a life well lived would need all the resources available to our multidisciplinary team and all of his willingness to take the help offered to him. And still, in the whole of his life story, so many questions remained unanswered.

Multidisciplinary Team (MDT) Care

Delivery of the best mental healthcare requires a team of professionals. Each example of modern therapy I have included in this book is delivered using a multidisciplinary approach. Each new care plan is introduced through the MDT and in each care plan the individual in distress is encouraged to work with its members. The strength of the therapeutic relationship is very important, so the challenge for any individual working in this MDT matrix is very great. It may not be easy for someone to establish and maintain the essential bonds of trust and kindness with a large group of people, and neither is it always easy for the team to respond to this challenge in a multilayered and skilled way.

Even still the MDT is the ideal vehicle of all modern healthcare. It is the cornerstone of every high-quality mental health service. It is not a formal therapy or even a particular style of practice; it is simply a group of people working together for the benefit of an individual in mental distress.

The ideal MDT includes a wide range of talents, assembled in a variety of ways depending on the clinical need. The standard team includes nurses, doctors and psychologists working with others, such as occupational therapists, social workers and psychotherapists. Obviously this complete tapestry of service provision is not available everywhere, but where it exists the MDT is by far and away the best method of delivering a complex, modern, effective care plan. No one human being can hope to bring all these required skills to the task of helping every patient on the road to recovery; this is why the MDT is best when it is diverse, skilled and coherent. Its leadership and its facilities need to be wide-ranging, and its work needs to be coherent, so as to unite around its common purpose: the restoration of a life well lived.

The MDT thrives in a therapeutic atmosphere of kindness and trust and, when it does this, something very special happens: genuine mental wellness and resilience begin to grow. Kindness enables the growth of this wellbeing. As we said earlier the ways to wellness (connection, learning, giving, taking notice and keeping active) can all expand if we are kind to ourselves and to each other.

The MDT rebuilds recovery and resilience by forming trust in its sincerity, in its expertise and ultimately in its therapy. Resilience grows on the same basis as trust, on a secure base, on education and on positive values. It expands in a setting of social competence and kinship, and requires a clinical vehicle with sufficient talent and interest to support each person in distress on their return to the life well lived. Put simply, the pathway to a life well lived is rebuilt by trust, kindness and teamwork.

Recovery as an Alternative to Stigma and Blame

Of all the responses to mental health difficulties, perhaps the most unhelpful response is 'blame'. At its worst blame is actually a form of stigma. We already know that harsh criticism is never useful, and yet we also know that 'pull yourself together' attitudes are the most common responses to mental distress. There may be some good reasons for frustration about those with mental health problems, but this is never therapeutic. It is common to hear people say that individuals in distress 'should just get on with things' and 'stop making such a fuss'. The effect of such dismissal is to make those already experiencing illness feel even more distressed and isolated. Pious admonishment does nothing to relieve the experience. Harsh judgement simply adds to suffering and exacerbates pain.

When mental health problems are judged in this way, a vicious cycle begins. When people in mental distress first seek help, they may be met with reassurance. Next comes advice. At this stage it is common to oversimplify mental health problems and this over-simplification leads many people to respond to mental distress by giving further advice. Unfortunately, this too may be experienced as yet another kind of dismissal – especially when those with enduring mental health difficulties are told to think more positively, to eat more sensibly, to take more exercise, to get better sleep, to be more mindful, and so on. This 'advice' is all very good and well intentioned, but the corollary needs to be acknowledged. Those who continue to experience mental health difficulties may be considered in some way to blame for their continuing problems. After all, as the logic goes, if they had taken sound advice, surely they would have overcome their problems by now.

In truth it is very difficult for most people to know what to do when they witness mental distress in others. Many family members feel helpless in this situation. So perhaps the first thing we could all do is to start by removing the word 'should' from our mental health vocabulary. The road to misery is paved with harsh judgement of others and also with harsh judgement of ourselves. Judging only adds to shame and frustration all around. To live life well again we would be well advised to stop 'should-ing' in our life. Each of us might try to live a day without saying 'you should', 'we should', 'they should' or even 'I should'. Imagine this, mind-fully. See how hard it would be, but also how liberating it might be. In the life well lived, no more 'should'!

It may not be easy to liberate ourselves in this way, but neither is it easy for those with mental health difficulties to overcome their self-reproach. In my experience, people in mental distress are the most critical of themselves, and their cycle of blame and shame is their most destructive problem of all. Critical judgements cast within mental health services are rarely, if ever, helpful or fair. Indeed, those criticized for their mental health problems are more often those who have been most disadvantaged from the start. Those blamed in mental healthcare are more likely to be women, children, the unemployed, the poor, the abused, the neglected, the migrant, or those already marginalized because of their race, colour or sexual orientation. Life includes many random factors. It seems achieving a well-lived life is like winning some kind of mental health lottery, but the opposite may also be true. Wellness is not absolute. It is relative, and recovery can be learned by any of us. The skills of recovery are transferable abilities and they are attributes that can be shared. Real recovery is about providing meaningful help and not judgemental guidance, however well intentioned.

Joseph's Journey Begins

Tuesday, 24 November 2015

Joseph speaks very softly during our conversation as a result of his Parkinson's disease. He is open about his life: there is much that remains still to be reconciled. Perhaps this is the root of his distress.

'My wife has been dead for nearly two years now. We were married for over thirty-five years, you know.'

'I'm very sorry to hear about your loss, Joseph. I really am. Were you and your wife—?'

'Phyllis.'

'Were you and Phyllis happy together, Joseph? A Darby and Joan couple?'

'Maybe. I was very lucky to have her. She was so kind to me. I miss her more each day.'

'And had Phyllis been sick for long?'

'Bone cancer. She had three years with it. We didn't heed the warnings. Left it too late, you know.'

'Her death must have left a huge void in your life.'

'It has, doctor, but she suffered, for sure, and she never complained – not once. She was a strong woman – a strong and loyal woman.'

'Loyal, you say?'

'Yes, loyal. She would never, over the years, give me any hassle, shall we say, over my crushes. She was very tolerant. I was actually always faithful to her, you know, but I did indulge in the odd bit of window shopping, if you know what I mean.'

'Right.'

'Forgive my voice, doctor. I got my diagnosis last year and I'm starting to see a dis-improvement recently. Damn thing.'

'It's Parkinson's disease, isn't it, Joseph?'

'Yes. Parkinson's.'

'And how are you coping with it?'

'Well, if I wasn't an old man before, I surely am now. I shuffle around like an old man, and I have this hand thing, like I'm *rolling a pill in my fingers*. Someone described it to me that way recently. And my voice is very soft. But otherwise it's . . . grand. If you know what I mean.'

'And so who is managing your Parkinson's?'

'I'm on some medication now, from my GP, but it's a progressive thing, as you can see. Parkinson's disease is something I am living with. I am becoming reconciled to it, even though the process of dying frightens me, Parkinson's disease doesn't frighten me. The depression is the worst of it all. It's what I fear more than anything.'

'Your GP is worried about you. He fears you may be close to total despair.'

'You mean he thinks that I might kill myself?'

'Is that on the cards, Joseph?'

'No, I don't think so. I have longed for death – to be with Phyllis. But I don't want to end my life that way. I am here today so that you will help me.'

'And I want to help you, Joseph, if that's what you want.'

256

'I want to make a fresh start. Even now, at this stage.'

'A fresh start? In what way would you like to make a fresh start, Joseph?'

'I suppose I should explain. Remember I told you about my *crushes*, as dear Phyllis used to call them?'

'You had an eye for the ladies, Joseph?'

'No, doctor. For the men.'

'The men?'

'Yes. I'm gay, doctor. I'm attracted to other men. All my life.'

'Oh, I see. Right.'

'Sorry to startle you, doctor.'

'No, no, not at all. Forgive me.'

'That's OK, doctor.'

'I understand.'

'I am not sure that you do!'

'Tell me then, did Phyllis know about your sexuality, Joseph?'

'Oh, yes. After all, we shared thirty-five years of marriage and the raising of our son. We had no secrets from each other. We loved each other dearly and we were each other's best friend.'

'And your son?'

'Simon.'

'And Simon, is he aware?'

'No, he doesn't know. We never saw the value in telling him.'

The unexpected turn in the conversation raises some questions: Why did Joseph and Phyllis marry all those years ago if he and Phyllis knew he was gay, and why did they stay together? Why was he still concealing his sexual orientation from his only son? Perhaps Joseph also felt this sense of confusion and it was linked to his depression.

'Maybe, doctor, things are different now. Maybe it's time for me to come out of the closet, or press, or whatever it is.'

'I think it's the closet.'

'Right – *closet*. Anyway, maybe I should be telling him now – telling other people too.'

'So, apart from Phyllis . . .'

'No one. Well, I've never openly broached it with anyone, not directly anyway.'

'Just Phyllis.'

'You see, with Phyllis I was so lucky. There was never a threat of her leaving me or anything like that. It was the opposite with her.'

'The opposite, Joseph? How would you describe that?'

'Well, she supported me, through everything, through all my bouts of depression she kept me going. I would not have got through my darkest days without her – not a hope.'

'And your depression today, would you say it's similar to previous episodes?'

'Similar, yes, but this time it seems even deeper and it's lasting much longer. Too long.'

'In what other ways is it different?'

'Over the years, I've had a few periods when my mood was low, but it always got better with time, and sometimes with prescribed help from a doctor. I need to take all the help I can get.'

'You have no objection to taking medication?'

'That's partly why I am here: I am hoping you will prescribe something powerful to lift my mood. I am a realist about treatment for this thing.'

'When was the last time your mood actually lifted?'

'Not since Phyllis's death. My form has not lifted at all.'

'Joseph, it would help me if you could tell me a bit more about your depression. Do you think you could describe a typical day for me?'

'Typical? Well, most mornings when I wake up I don't want to get up. Facing the day becomes utter torture. I can see no future. It is as if nothing is visible. I lie awake most nights.'

'I imagine your Parkinson's doesn't help either.'

'Yes, the shaking alone makes it hard to sleep.'

'So are you exhausted the next day?'

'The rest of the day is such a struggle. I haven't any energy. I've no concentration and no appetite. I'm down 10 kilos since

Phyllis . . . And as you can see, I don't need to lose any weight.'

'So you reckon you are depressed?'

'After all this time, doctor, I can recognize it. I understand depression. I know the gloom and the paralysing feeling. All too well. All too often.'

'You have had more than your fair share of blows over the past few years, with your bereavement and now this neurological diagnosis. This would be very hard on any person, Joseph.'

'There have been good times and some heavy blows, but the depression – and the shame of it – is by far the worst thing. It's invisible and unspeakable. It's even worse than the grief over Phyllis's death.'

'Can you distinguish your grief from your depression, Joseph?'

'I don't mean to sound callous, doctor – but in some ways, I am actually glad she has gone. She might have had a very hard time, except that the hospice was so good. I know she is happy now. We both believe in Paradise, you know?'

'Paradise?'

'Yes, we had strong faith.'

There is a brief pause in the conversation at this point. Joseph takes a moment to collect his thoughts.

'Have you felt under pressure because you are gay, Joseph – perhaps the pressure of keeping it secret for all those years?'

'No, not at all. I was born gay. I'm not ashamed of that. I don't feel guilty for being gay, if that's what you're getting at.'

'No, Joseph, don't get me wrong, I'm not saying that. But I thought that maybe there has been some religious pressure to conceal that part of your life.'

'Why do you ask that?'

'Well, you told me that you and Phyllis believed in Paradise, is that correct?'

'Yes, we did. I do.'

'So, I take it that you and Phyllis were, for want of a better phrase, regular church goers, Joseph?'

'Look, it's not as simple as that. I have my faith. I believe in God and I believe God loves me. God made me, and he made me gay. I believe God loves me for who I am. God loves me and so God loves me gay. Anyway, there it is: God loves me. Do you understand what I am saying? Maybe I'm not making any sense.'

'Yes, you are, Joseph. You are making sense – perfect sense . . . Has your faith ever been a source of consolation to you, Joseph?'

'Yes, it has been. It was something Phyllis and I could share. We were in a prayer group together, in our parish. Since her death, the others have tried to be good to me. They knew Phyllis well but, to tell you the truth, it's not the same for me without her.'

'Depression can make faith hard.'

'No, it's not just my faith that suffers. It's my prayers. They are very hard. When I pray, I have a conversation with God and I know I am in his company. But there is the problem: when I am depressed, I cannot speak. It's as if the depression steals my words and my happiness. My prayers will not come to me, and so I feel utterly cut off. My prayers are unborn.'

'Have you been able to continue to go to the prayer group?'

'Not as often, but now and again. Like I said, it's not the same without Phyllis. I don't look for sympathy, doctor, but that's all I seem to get now with the group. Don't get me wrong, they're trying to, I suppose, console me. But I know that's not what I need right now.'

'And what is it you feel that you need at this time, Joseph?'

'Well, some help from you, for a start. In the past, a prescription has helped to lift my mood. I think I'll need something a little stronger this time, though.'

'And is there anything else you need?'

'Yes, I need your psychological help too. Like I say, I know you can do something more than give me pills.'

'Absolutely, Joseph, I can. If you are willing to work with me.'

'Yes, this is my last hope, doctor.'

Thursday, 17 December 2015

Joseph returns. We talk about how his medication is working and if it is relieving his distress. Joseph talks some more about his relationship with Phyllis and his son Simon.

'And how do you feel today, Joseph?'

'The Parkinson's? I try not to think too much about it. Obviously I can't avoid the visible problems. I don't like being stared at.'

'Do people stare?'

'Ah, I can see, sometimes on the bus or in the supermarket. Children mostly.'

'Well, from my point of view, Joseph, you look very well today – considering all you are dealing with.'

'I was in the queue at the post office – yesterday, I think. And a little girl, looking back over her mother's shoulder said, "Mammy, what's wrong with that old man's hands?"'

'Oh dear.'

'Yes, I know. She was just a little girl: she didn't mean anything by it. But it was the look of embarrassment and sympathy on her mother's face, when she turned to me. I don't want to be . . . well, I suppose I don't want to stand out. I never have. Do you understand, doctor?'

'Yes, I do, Joseph.'

'The worst thing is, before, I had Phyllis. She was like my shield for society.'

'How so?'

'Well, I felt protected. She was like a forcefield. She gave me strength and confidence. I'm exposed now – vulnerable and not just 'cause of my sexuality.'

'Can you explain that to me?'

'It's the stigma, I suppose. I always knew I could be marked out. Phyllis was my minder in more ways than one: being gay, being depressed.'

'Talk to me a little bit more about your life with Phyllis. What else did you have in common?'

'We had lots in common. We were a team, a good team. We did everything together. We both really enjoyed going to shows and whenever we could travel abroad we liked to see a show and visit the great museums. We loved paintings – just beautiful things in general. Beautiful things always lifted me. Phyllis knew that.'

'And your son, Simon, where is he now?'

'Do you have children, doctor?'

'Yes, I do.'

'You know the way people talk about parenthood: "Nobody tells you how hard it is"?'

'Yes, I've heard that said.'

'Well, I never got that. For me, parenthood was a joy, and for Phyllis as well. She was such a great mother, and still is. She will always be a great mother. That's one type of eternity.'

'You sound like you both really enjoyed raising your son, watching him grow up. Did you ever consider having more children?'

'No. One was it for us. He is a good one.'

'Is Simon still living near?'

'No, he got an opportunity to study his music in Rome a few years ago. Once in a lifetime opportunity. We were so proud of his talent.'

'Oh, that's fantastic.'

'He worked so hard at it, hour after hour, when all the other kids were playing football or whatever. Phyllis and I loved music, but neither of us could hold a note, never mind play a Bach suite. But Simon – now he is quite the musician.'

'You're very proud of Simon.'

'Couldn't be prouder of him. Couldn't be prouder.'

'And you miss him?'

'Yes, of course. But he has to follow his star. We all have to follow our own star. I'm a real believer in that. But I do miss the sound of him practising, his music echoing through the house. It brought life and art into our home. It's a wonderful thing, you know?'

'Yes, I do know.'

'Anyway, he calls me every other day, ever since his mother died. He really does care. He's a good son.'

'Tell me, Joseph, do you feel that you have a star of your own to follow?'

'Possibly, but I feel . . . I feel my star is fading. Maybe my star is burning out. They all do in the end, you know.'

'Yes, but they shouldn't before their time, don't you think?'

'I know what you're saying, doctor, but every time I have this battle, to come out of a dark place, it takes more effort. And I'm getting weaker.'

'We can work together on your strength, Joseph. Are the tablets I gave you last time starting to help?'

'Not yet, as far as I can tell. You did say it might take a couple of weeks before I noticed any improvement.'

'Yes, that's true. And in the meantime, what helps you to carry on?'

'Two things have helped me to get out of these black holes in the past: kindness and beauty.'

'So do you seek out beautiful things when you're low – to lift you?'

'Yes, exactly. But I had Phyllis's help in the past. She supplied the kindness, which in turn enabled me to find the beauty – in the world, in people, in art, in music . . . Do you understand?'

Joseph begins to weep now. He sits for a moment lost in his thoughts.

'Joseph, would you like a tissue? I hope I didn't upset you in any way . . .'

'No, no, doctor. I'll be fine.'

'We can always talk again, at another time, if you don't feel up to it today.'

'Please, let's go on, doctor.'

'Certainly, if you want to, Joseph.'

'These Parkinson's pills make my mouth dry. Sometimes it's hard to talk.'

'Here, have some water, Joseph.'

'Thank you, doctor. I haven't spoken like this for a long time, not really since Phyllis died.'

'It's good that you can talk this way, Joseph. I am sorry for upsetting you.'

'You're not upsetting me, you know. I want to be well again. Depression makes me feel cut off from everyone and everything. Talking means reconnecting and that's healing for me. I don't talk about my depression with anyone.'

'Joseph, did you always know that you were gay?'

'That's right.'

'Yet you still married Phyllis.'

'Yes.'

'If you don't mind my asking – why? If you knew you were gay.'

'Doctor, I'm here for your help. I trust you – I have to – but I must request one thing, one very important thing from you.'

'Yes, of course, Joseph, what would that be?'

'Don't judge me too harshly.'

'Forgive me, Joseph, I was not judging you at all – nor would I ever. I promise you that.'

'The last thing I need right now, doctor, is to be burdened with the attitudes of today.'

'I hope I would never do that. That's not how we work, Joseph.'

'Look, doctor, the sexual issue seems academic to me now. Being gay, or straight for that matter, is not all about sexual acts. That's where people have it wrong: it's not about what I do, it's about who I am. Do you understand that?'

'I do understand, Joseph. And Phyllis understood that too?'

'*Voilà*. Now you know why I married her.'

'Right, but you did want to marry her, didn't you?'

'Back in those days, things were very different. If you were twenty and there was no sign of a girlfriend, people began to wonder about you. *Pig's-ear, Nancy boy* – all of that stuff. But I really loved Phyllis and I loved being married to her.'

'And what about your sexuality?'

'I tried to suppress or ignore it at first, and as the years went by it became more and more difficult for me. This can't be that unusual. Believe me, lots of gay men are married to women, and lots of gay women are married to men. But back then nobody ever talked about being gay. There was no *coming out*.'

'OK, Joseph, I understand.'

'I see the gay pride parades today and it gives me a great lift, a bit of faith in humanity. But back then, well, let's just say if there had been a gay pride parade, we'd have been lucky not to be lynched!'

'It can't have been easy for either of you. So my question remains, why, do you think, did Phyllis agree to marry you? Knowing everything.'

'Do you not think Phyllis could have loved a gay man?'

'Forgive me, Joseph, that's not what I meant at all. But can you see what I'm getting at? Understanding why people choose to come together and why they stay together is a mystery, but I reckon it involves more than just an assumption that they were in love.'

'Phyllis had her challenges too, without a doubt, but we were best of friends from the time we met. And we were getting closer, and then when Phyllis got pregnant . . . well, that kind of sealed it for me. I was staying. I was happy.'

'They were good years for you?'

'I think my best. And Simon, well, from day one I raised him like he was my own flesh and blood.'

'Your own flesh and blood?'

'Yes. Obviously I'm not Simon's biological father.'

'Oh.'

'Well, myself and Phyllis . . . in the beginning we were just good friends, as they say. Then she became pregnant.'

'So, do you mind if I ask, was she seeing someone else at the time?'

'Yes, and he left her high and dry!'

'But you weren't OK with that, Joseph?'

'Look, doctor, back then things would have been really difficult for a single mother. So we got married. Sure, Phyllis and I didn't have a conventional marriage, but it worked for us. It worked very well. I told you not to judge me.'

'Oh, I'm not judging – just trying to understand.'

'No, when it happened, Phyllis confided in me and I offered to marry her at once. Like I said, we were a team.'

'OK, well, that's taken me a little by surprise. I assumed Simon was your—'

'He is mine, doctor. I raised him from day one with Phyllis and I love him very much, as he loves me.'

'And is Simon aware of his . . .'

'Yes, we told him as soon as was appropriate, and asked him if he wanted to have a relationship with his biological father.'

'And did he want that?'

'He's a bright boy. He said maybe, if and when he feels the time is right.'

'And the time is not right yet?'

'It's his call. Completely. We were all agreed on that. He's a smart boy. I trust his judgement.'

'And do you know who Simon's biological father is, Joseph?'

'I know of him. We've never spoken, but he's an old work colleague of Phyllis. He was a good-looking man. I could see why she was attracted to him.'

'And your partnership with Phyllis worked out.'

'That's right. It worked out, and you said it, we were our own Darby and Joan couple.'

Tuesday, 12 January 2016

Joseph's health seems to be improving, however we discuss the possibility of him coming and staying in hospital for a few days so that the combination of his medications and treatment can be rebalanced.

'Have you been able to do any of the things that you love since Phyllis's passing, Joseph?'

'Well, recently I've been feeling a bit better. My sleep is no better, but the mornings have lifted a bit. I expect the medication is kicking in.'

'Yes, but you've more than one problem to contend with, of course.'

'Yes, my Parkinson's still makes things more difficult.'

'What kind of things, Joseph?'

'Lots of things. Sleeping or travelling anywhere, or being independent. But, anyway, I don't want to go abroad – or anywhere, really.'

'And there are things of beauty closer to home – here in Dublin.'

'Oh, of course, I know. Sure, I used to spend hours sitting in front of the Vermeer in the National Gallery. Or the Velázquez – wonderful works. Do you know Vermeer's *Lady Writing a Letter with Her Maid*?'

'Sure.'

'After Vermeer died, his wife used it to pay the local baker to cover a bill. Did you know that, doctor?'

'No, I didn't know that. That's incredible.'

'Yes – and Velázquez, *Kitchen Maid*? You know the one with the Last Supper in the background. Ah, it's fascinating.'

'I can see that even talking about these beautiful things lifts your spirits, Joseph.'

'Yes, it does, but I just didn't have the . . . will, or the energy before. I'm trying to find that strength again. But it's hard for me to get even a few hours' sleep at night with the new medications you gave me.'

'How are you finding them?'

'OK, like I said. But I wish I was getting a bit of sleep.'

'Joseph, would you consider coming in here to the hospital with us for a couple of nights?'

'You're not trying to lock me up, I hope.'

'No, not at all. You see, I've been talking with your medical team and your GP and we all agree that it is vital that the combination of your medications and your treatment is rebalanced. We have to be mindful of the risks of interactions and side effects and all that goes with this territory.'

'I want to understand, doctor. It's not what I had planned . . . but if you think it's necessary I'll come in. But for how long? I can't stay too long, you know.'

'It will be just for a few days, maybe a week, if you are willing to stay?'

'OK. OK, yes. I'll come in. I can hear Phyllis's voice in my head already. She always encouraged me to be decisive.'

'That's great, Joseph, but it's not just about balancing the medication. If you are happy, we can work together with our team of nurses and our neurologist. You could also use the help of a physiotherapist and occupational therapist, to help with your mobility, so you can get around easier.'

'They can do all this in a couple of days? I doubt it.'

'No, not quite. But it would be an introduction to them and an intensive start to this kind of team treatment. And of course you can follow up later with the rest of the team as a day-patient in our Wellness and Recovery Centre. Trust me, it's what we call the multidisciplinary approach. Joseph, this could open up a world of remedies for you. The team are fantastic at what they do.'

'Well, I'm not jumping for joy about this, doctor. But I have decided to do whatever it takes to get well. It's not just that I have Phyllis in my head telling me to get on with it.'

'What is it, then?'

'It's that I have decided to be here for me and for Simon. I am here, for real. I want to make the best of what is left for me – whatever it takes.'

'And you can, Joseph. I'll check in regularly, as often as you want. There is a lot more for us to talk about, isn't there?'

'Yes. I do still want to talk. There is more I want to talk to you about.'

'Good, Joseph. That's what I am here for.'

'I'll have to get someone to mind the house. Oh, and the cat. I'll have to get someone to feed the cat. He's on medication too, would you believe? Poor old Sour Puss. Phyllis said she named him after me!'

'She had a good sense of humour, then?'

'Yes, really great, actually. I had the sour puss.'

'Do you have neighbours, maybe, or family to help?'

'My neighbours are really good people. I'll get Joe next door to do it. I'll tell him I'm just going in for a little procedure. I don't want them knowing. It's nobody's business. I don't want to be talking about it. I'll make up something about a procedure. Yes, that's what I'll do.'

'OK, Joseph, it is such a good idea to take time to organize things. That way you won't have to worry about anything. We can help you to get it organized, if you like?'

'No, no, it's not that much. I'll be OK. Is next week too soon?'

'No, the sooner the better. I'll make the arrangements this end. Joseph, we have more time today, if you wish to talk some more?'

'No, no, I'll go and get started. Sure, I can talk to you next week, can't I? When I'm in here.'

'Absolutely, Joseph.'

'Well, I'd better go, get on with it, like I said. I'd better let Simon know, tell him not to worry.'

'Have you seen much of Simon recently?'

'He's due back for a visit in a couple of months, so I'll tell him not to come before then. No need.'

'Joseph, the team will take great care of you. I promise.'

Tuesday, 22 March 2016

Two months have passed since our last meeting. Following his hospital stay, Joseph now meets regularly with the multidisciplinary team. He discusses how he is using acceptance in his treatment. Simon, his son, will be home to visit in a week and Joseph is preparing for his arrival.

'Joseph, it's great to see you again. You look really well.'

'Thank you, doctor. Yes, I'm feeling a bit better. I think my star is starting to burn a little brighter.'

'And how do you feel your sessions are going with the team? They tell me that you are doing exceptionally well.'

'Exceptionally? I don't know really. I'd say "good". I'm glad I agreed to come in. And I'm glad to come in to the recovery centre every week, it is helping me.'

'It's been a couple of months now, hasn't it? Do you feel differently at all?'

'You mean mentally or physically?'

'Well, both actually. They go better together.'

'You're right there, doctor. The physio is really good. I thought I would just get worse and worse with the mobility, but I see an improvement, especially in the early part of the day. The guys in the clinic were saying that's typical enough, but they say that I can improve further, so I'm sticking with it.'

'And your mood, Joseph, it seems to have lifted?'

'I know, it has lifted. It's hard to tell by how much. I mean, when you're down, sometimes you don't know just how down you are. But I know that I'm going in the right direction. I'm getting good signs.'

'"Good signs", Joseph – how do you mean?'

'Well, it doesn't take a genius to tell, especially if you've been down there before. I've lots of experience of the blues.'

'And what would be the main improvements you are seeing, Joseph?'

'Better sleep, for sure. My Parkinson's is better controlled as well, so I'm not as restless at night. I'm better able for your "Eyes open, feet on the floor" drill. Thanks for that one, by the way. It's quite effective, you know?'

'Well, I'm glad to hear it, Joseph.'

'Also my appetite – it's coming back. Before I just had no interest in eating. Now I think I've put on a bit of weight. I'm certainly not losing any more anyway.'

'Good, this is great to hear.'

'Look, I know I'm not going to get rid of the Parkinson's, but I am surprised how much it can improve, with the work we're doing.'

'Good, and the team tell me that you're giving it everything you've got. It's a courageous thing to do, Joseph. It's not easy.'

'It's like I said, doctor. I am here for real. Do you understand?'

'Of course I do. That's the reason you have improved. Nothing would have changed without you entering into the spirit of recovery.

Nothing would have changed unless you wanted to do this.'

'You know, my physiotherapist said something to me the other day that really lifted me. It struck a chord.'

'What was that, Joseph?'

'She told me to look at my problems and accept them as "my own". They are about me and within me. They're OK. They are mine.'

'Does she want you to be more mindful?'

'Yes, I suppose she does, whatever that means. There has been a lot of talk in the team about being mindful.'

'So, how does that help?'

'Well, for me it's like a mantra, like "acceptance" I suppose. I think I accept my problems are in me, but I also have to accept that the same is true for the solutions. It's OK to search within myself for my solutions.'

'And when you search for solutions, Joseph, where are you beginning to find them?'

'Now that I am feeling better, living well has become possible. I am not saying it's easy. But the alternative is worse – much worse. I have been struggling for so long, always looking for solutions from outside, and whenever I look inward it only leads to more blame and shame.'

'There is no joy in either of those, Joseph.'

'No, I thought I was finished, you know, I really did. But now I feel there might be a little spark. There is hope. Maybe my star's not ready to burn out just yet.'

'Absolutely, Joseph.'

'Who was it, doctor, the guy who said it's better to burn out than to fade away? I can't remember . . . But anyway, I'm not sure I fully agree with that now.'

'Indeed, you might have something there, Joseph. And how are you coping with everything at home?'

'Well, now I have the home care to check in on me once a week. It's great. I feel I'll probably need it more in the future, but I appreciate it even now. She's a lovely young lady, a nurse – full of life. It's good for the house too, you know? Another heartbeat around the place.'

'Yes, that is good. And there's also your cat. Sour Puss, I believe you called him.'

'Ha! Yeah, Sour Puss is hanging in there, like myself. He's getting on too. I might have to start bringing him in here with me! Home is definitely a little brighter. I still miss Phyllis so much, but I'm starting to get used to living without her.'

'And Simon, how is he?'

'He's coming next week to stay with me, for two weeks. I am so looking forward to that. He worries, you know?'

'Yes, and he's lost his mother too.'

'He adored her, and she adored him. I get so low, sometimes, I forget that. I can see that today. I want to be able to talk to him about her and not just pull the covers over my head at the thought of it.'

'So, you feel good talking to Simon about her?'

'About her, and me, and him. Depression strangles the life out of these things. I have to fight it. I am fighting, for Simon's sake.'

'And your own, Joseph?'

'Yes, and for my own sake. I know what Phyllis would say. I know what she would want. I want to make her proud.'

At this point tears well up in Joseph's eyes. He takes a moment to compose his thoughts.

'I'm not sad, doctor, just sometimes I pine for the way things were, you know, with Phyllis?'

'I understand, Joseph, never forget the happy times you had with her.'

'You're right, and we'll always be soulmates. I've started to talk to her again, you know, at night if I can't sleep. I used to pray, or talk to God, I suppose. I do want to get back to doing that, definitely. But in the meantime she is my go-between. I'm still angry – not as angry as before – but I'm still a little angry with God for taking her away from me. But I have faith in Phyllis. I always did.'

'And the talking helps you, Joseph?'

'Yes, helps me sleep. I don't feel as abandoned.'

'Do you feel Phyllis abandoned you?'

'No, but I feel life did, there, for a while. Maybe it's coming back.'

'Simon's company will be nice for you.'

'Yes, we haven't really spoken about Phyllis properly. I mean, we talk every other day – chit-chat, how's the weather in Rome, that sort of thing – but we haven't *spoken* about her.'

'And you – you could speak about yourself and Simon, and your future?'

'Yes, I suppose so, doctor. We do have a future to talk about.'

'Are you still able to get out and about, Joseph?'

'I am, a little – just locally now. But I do want to get into the National Gallery again. I read about an exhibition that I'd love to see, maybe with Simon.'

'Sounds like a beautiful day out, Joseph.'

'Yes, maybe. And I'm going to tell him.'

'Tell him? What are you going to tell him?'

'I'm going to tell him I'm gay. I've decided. I ran it by Phyllis the other night in my mind and sure I knew what she would say.'

'This is good, Joseph. Simon sounds like an intelligent young man, so I'm sure he'll understand why you didn't tell him before now.'

'Well, it's not that straightforward, doctor. It's a big secret to keep from your son for all these years.'

'But now's a good time to tell him, I would think, Joseph.'

'But I am ashamed. I feel I failed him.'

'How so?'

'Well, when Simon was at college, in his first year, he brought home a boyfriend.'

'Right. So Simon is also gay?'

'Yes, of course. Did I not mention that?'

'No, I don't think you did. So I assume you had no issues with Simon's sexuality, Joseph?'

'Of course not. But I didn't exactly embrace it, or support it, maybe, quite as much as I should. All things considered.'

'OK, so maybe now's a better time, Joseph?'

'I hope he understands. Nobody understood more than me what he was going through. And yet I kind of clammed up. I froze. Stigma, I suppose. I didn't want him to judge me and to find me wanting.'

'I understand that, Joseph.'

'The three "S"s, doctor. We were talking about it in one of my sessions a few weeks ago: stigma, shame and secrets. A nasty little triangle. Each one feeds the other and they starve everything else. Do you know what I mean?'

'Yes, I do. I understand completely.'

'But I'm going to try and put it right with Simon.'

'Well, you have a perfect opportunity to do so.'

'I hope he understands.'

Tuesday, 26 April 2016

Joseph's physical and mental health are steadily improving. He is working closely with the multidisciplinary team, focusing on bringing balance into his life. He feels positive about his recovery and his future.

'Good to see you again, Joseph. You look well. How have things been with you since we last talked?'

'I feel well, maybe. Certainly better than before. Let's say I'm heading in the direction of well.'

'That's great to hear.'

'I can see steady progress in my mobility. I'm getting around a lot easier. It's amazing how we take our mobility for granted.'

'Yes, Joseph, and being unable to get around can have a huge effect on our mental wellbeing.'

'Yes, I can see that now. I took my mobility for granted when I was younger. What is it the song says? *You don't know what you've got till it's gone.*'

'Indeed, we see that all the time here in our clinics. Physical health is so important to your mental health and vice versa.'

'Yes, Trish, the nurse in the clinic, is great. She really keeps me on my toes, so to speak. I think I actually enjoy the workout.'

'Trish is great, one of our best trainers. We call what she does behavioural activation.'

'Getting going? It's good. I suppose I'm working out a lot of things. I thought I was beyond that sort of thing, an old guy like me.'

'We're never too old to improve our health – both mental and physical.'

'Yes, I believe that now. I actually do. It's funny, I was thinking about it on the bus the other day. I saw a guy outside a pub in town, middle of the day, middle of the week, and he was having a go at passers-by, just completely out of control.'

'Right.'

'I mean, really having a go: shouting and waving his arms. Distressed, you know, really distressed. I felt for him, poor guy, and I thought: there is a guy that needs to get control of himself.'

'And this got you thinking about yourself, Joseph?'

'Yes. It came to me: I've always had such control, always, saw it as a good thing. Always in control, maybe over-controlled, no matter what. In control of my expressions, my emotions, the whole lot.'

'And now you see it differently?'

'Yes, I am learning to let go of the control from time to time. It was a light bulb moment, doctor, you know?'

'I do, Joseph.'

'I'm sure your team have been patiently bringing me around to this point, but you have to see it yourself for it to . . . click, you know?'

'I agree, Joseph. These moments we have – on the bus, chopping vegetables for dinner, driving around – wherever these moments happen, they can be big moments in our lives.'

'Yeah, I know it's never going to make the papers – "Old Man On Bus Has Revelation!" – but it's big for me.'

'Of course, Joseph, absolutely. Recovery of life rarely makes the papers these days, unfortunately.'

'Yes, I've stopped reading them. Don't get me wrong, it's not that I don't care – I don't want to lose touch – but I can do without all the doom and gloom. It's not good for the head.'

'So let's go back to your control revelation, Joseph. I'm interested to hear more.'

'Well, that's it really. As I said, I always thought control was a positive, never even gave that a second thought. Now I see it can be a negative too. I suppose too much control of anything is not good. I'm trying to get more of a balance. I don't want to swing too far the other way, you know?'

'Yes, indeed. So many of these things are about our balance. I often meet people who have to learn about balance: everyone needs a little more of that.'

'Yes, I can see all these little things – all the pieces, pieces of a puzzle.'

'That's it, Joseph. All of these little "revelations". They are so vital for us.'

'Yes, I get that now.'

'Tell me, Joseph. Did Simon come to visit? We were talking about his visit the last time?'

'He did. He was only meant to stay for two weeks. I think he stayed nearly four. He stayed with me in the house.'

'And you enjoyed his company?'

'Oh, yes. We had a good time. He's actually moving back permanently in a couple of months – once he passes his latest exams, of course. But I have no worries there. He's never failed an exam in his life. I think he'll be one of those guys who is still doing exams – and doing well at them – into old age. So yes, he's moving back.'

'Great, and he'll be nearby when he returns?'

'Very nearby. He's going to move back in, would you believe? Just until he gets on his feet here. Have you seen the price of rent around our area?'

'Yes, I have. It's very difficult for people to find a decent, affordable place.'

'Yes, it's just awful, but I'm not complaining. I'll take the company, and I'm glad I have something to offer him, to help him out. He says he wants to be here.'

'And we talked, Joseph, at the last session, about you having a conversation with Simon, do you recall?'

'Yes, I do – of course.'

'And did it go the way you had hoped?'

'Well, we were sitting in the National Gallery, enjoying *The Taking of Christ* – the Caravaggio – you know it?'

'I do, of course. It is wonderful.'

'Absolutely mesmerizing. I just love it. Anyway, we were there, it was midweek, early enough. We were the only ones there and I thought, OK, now's the time.'

'So you told him?'

'Oh, sure, I should have known not to worry when it comes to Simon. Do you know what he said to me when I told him? When I told him I was gay? My big dark secret?'

'No, what did he say?'

'He said, "Ah, Dad, tell me something I don't know, will you?" Just like that. Just like we were shooting the breeze. Can you believe it?'

'So, he wasn't upset?'

'No! He told me he'd known a long time. He said something to me, and it made me cry – tears of joy – relief, maybe. But he said that when he came out and told us, Phyllis and I, that I told him with my eyes. I told him with my eyes that I loved him and that I was gay too. So all this time he knew.'

'But he never said.'

'He never said. I asked him, why didn't you say? He just said he felt it was never the right time. He said it was a conversation that I needed to start.'

'You were concerned about his reaction?'

'Yes, and I need not have been.'

'So where is your relationship now . . . with Simon?'

'Well, that was the last of the secrets – gone in a puff of smoke. Good riddance. You know we talked so much, and not just "weather" stuff. We talked about Phyllis. We laughed and cried about her, sometimes at the same time. It was a healing time for us: nobody loved her as much as we did.'

'Sometimes, Joseph, talking and listening to each other is all the healing that you need at that moment.'

'Yes. Real talking. Honest talking. Simon is coming out of a relationship himself, he is quite down about it actually. But, you know, I think I can help him. He's told me all about it and I think that our talking helped him too. Imagine that: the old closet gay helping the young proud gay son!'

'This life and learning is so valuable, Joseph, to you and your son. We learn more from our experiences when we are willing to pay attention to them. Do you know what I mean?'

'I do now, doctor. And I'm still learning.'

Joseph's Journey

Sometimes even a well-lived life needs mending. Our hearts break and when they do our minds break down for a time and we need mending. Sometimes recovery is about acknowledging our need for repair. People and things fall apart, but when they do, therapy can bring individuals in distress together again. Since mental distress is about disintegration of the mind and the body, recovery is about restoring wholeness.

This is the value of mental healthcare. All modern therapies are about this same purpose. They aim to reunite the mind with the body, physical energy with the spirit. This restoration of human integrity requires teamwork. To be effective we need to bring together many insights and therapeutic skills to assist those whose expertise has been acquired through painful experience of distress.

Listening to people in this therapeutic way means hearing them and valuing their perspective. This was true for Joseph's therapy and it is true for the health service as a whole. After a bad experience in mental healthcare some people feel like the proverbial 'canary in the mineshaft', as if the 'system' were happy for them to expire, if only as a warning to others. Our systems also need to change. We need to listen. We need to provide genuine multidisciplinary therapy for people whose problems are complex. If we continue to ignore individual concerns, including the demand for better and more effective therapy, sooner or later there will be no therapeutic mental healthcare available at all. We will be left with little actual healthcare apart from institutional reviews and governance reports written after the events. Although heard by endless commissions of inquiry, these are mostly ignored by real human beings.

So, is Joseph well now? It's true, Joseph has experienced many aspects of healthcare, and not just one specific psychotherapy. His treatment has followed a shared multidisciplinary care plan, and that treatment was given in an atmosphere of mindfulness, respect and kindness. Throughout his journey Joseph engaged with supportive care in a trusting therapeutic relationship backed up by a multidisciplinary team with skills in nursing, neurology, pharmacology, psychology and physiotherapy. In short, he had a full mental health service team.

Each intervention focused on a particular problem. His needs determined his care. Nothing more. Nothing less. But each intervention was joined up to the others by way of the team. What emerged was an integrated MDT care plan. Joseph's care plan brought medicine of the mind and body together in order to bring his mental and physical health together. His care plan addressed a wide range of problems, a list as wide as his humanity itself. Obviously these problems included Joseph's recurring depression, his Parkinson's disease, his grief and his experience of stigma relating to his sexuality. He was also coming to terms with changes in his personal circumstances and in his relationship with his son. These issues required an even deeper engagement. That may be why his care was effective. But that is what is so rewarding about mental healthcare: seeing recovery and believing it is possible. Recovery of a life well lived is about women and men being given the opportunity to fully engage in the process of achieving wellness.

Today, Joseph's depression has lifted and his neurological condition has improved to such a degree that he is more mobile and outgoing. He is much better able to sleep and to travel. Indeed, since his recovery he has travelled with Simon to many places. His physical and mental health have become more integrated and they have progressed together. So, yes, I would say that Joseph is much improved. But there is more still.

Now Joseph has a recovery plan that he can follow. His initial recovery was possible because he was able to be truly present and so he fully engaged in this recovery process. He was willing to search for solutions from both outside and within himself. He has also become more mindful, and his stress levels have reduced.

So you may ask: What about other things, the realities that neither he nor any of us can change? What about death and dying? How it is possible to live well when someone has such a long history of secrecy and denial? There was no escaping his recent bereavement from his wife Phyllis, and he must face the many challenges in the future with his physical health.

Mindfulness played its part and so it turns out that Joseph's view has changed. He accepts the realities of his past, and despite everything he feels sure that he is in a better place today. Nothing can bring the dead back to life – Joseph knows that. But because of his genuine presence and engagement in his recovery he has been able to do something really special, perhaps an especially mindful thing each of us needs to do: he has been able to engage with help and work towards recovery. Now he is living in the present. There will be no more hiding. Now, with the team's help and with his son, Joseph's health can grow and he can experience wellness again, for however long remains for him. Joseph has found the ability to seize the day and to make himself available for new opportunities in the future. Joseph has recovered hope and that has always been part of what it takes to live life well.

New Paths to a Life Well Lived

Throughout this book we have been considering the true meaning of 'wellness' and highlighting some hopeful developments and new ways of restoring mental health. We have journeyed together on a number of different paths to a well-lived life. Hopefully this personal witness of recovery has been as compelling for you as it has been for me. Here is the proof of the pudding we have been looking for. It is to be found daily in the lives of countless numbers of people who have lost their mental health and then rediscovered it through the experience of modern therapy. So, how can this recovery be sustained and how can access to it be widened?

I hope you will agree that modern therapy needs to be made more available, more affordable, and also more reliable. These three agendas are service questions often obscured in this area by institutional debates about history, politics and health economics. These are important concerns, but even these topics fail to address the most important human issues at stake in therapy. To discover what matters for individual human beings in therapy we cannot avoid one crucial question: What is it that makes a therapeutic relationship successful? By comparison to our usual health service debate this issue may seem small, but it is actually very important. The answer to *this* question may be the key to the delivery of effective mental healthcare.

Communication in therapy is private and personal and sometimes painful. Desires common to us all and present in all our intimate relationships underpin much of this special dialogue. Conscious and unconscious elements are always active. A therapeutic relationship is special. It is always human, and so while it is universal it is unique at the same time. Within this protean landscape two issues are recurrent and both are of critical importance to the effectiveness of therapy. First, there is the necessity for 'trust', and second there is the need for 'kindness'. These two powerful dynamics actually determine the 'success' or 'failure' of any therapy and so we need to value them far more than we do. We need to see trust and kindness as essential clinical assets and also as human rights. Those with mental health difficulties return to these issues, in some form or other, again and again and again. If we listen carefully, we hear these concerns. So, what can we do about them?

Trust in Healthcare

Trust is the essential prescription for our health service. The evidence is that trust in health services has been declining for many years, but this decline has been steepest in mental healthcare. The 'psych wars' we mentioned earlier came upon the background of undeniable failures in the nineteenth- and twentieth-century asylum system. To my mind our preoccupation with the ghoulish history of 'psychiatry' has reached worrying proportions. The future demands a repaired vision of psychiatry. We need to replace this history with a more inclusive vision of our mental healthcare system. Without sufficient belief in the future of mental healthcare we will inevitably return to our painful past. Sadly, our collective disappointment with the 'system' of psychiatry has yet to be mitigated by much success from the new systems of 'care in the community'. Arresting the decline of trust in our mental health services will not be easy. Trust that 'is built upon many steps may be destroyed in one'.[1]

Restoring trust in mental healthcare is still possible. It is essential. Better mental health is part of the solution for all our health services and this new prescription is *not* just about

---

[1] Quote from Eric Hoffer in David A. Shore, *The Trust Prescription for Healthcare: Building Your Reputation with Consumers*, Health Administration Press, 2011.

psychiatry. Modern mental healthcare is inclusive of all disciplines and of many different skill sets. This multidisciplinary vision means integrating psychiatry with psychology, nursing, social work and occupational therapy and also the service user. If we leave anything or anyone out of the sum, the whole will be damaged.

We have a shared goal, so this teamwork makes sense. Our pursuit of wellness is about everyone and not just for a minority. Our shared vision of a life well lived is about people getting better and not just better-off. To achieve this renewed vision our mental healthcare system will need to be 'trusted'. To earn this trust, our mental healthcare services will need to be different from the 'psychiatry' of the past. We will need to be effective and coherent with human rights. This new mental healthcare will be about community care because it reliably returns human beings to communities that care.

The caring community also deserves to know that a modern and effective mental healthcare system is worth the investment. That is one reason why education about mental healthcare is so important. As ever, society can have no health until it restores our mental health. A more effective mental healthcare system could be provided on the basis of evidence, on the principles of justice and on a platform of prudent investment. And this investment would not just be about money. We could restore trust in the mental health services by investing in mutual respect – in each other, in the science of our methods, and in the human rights of those we serve.

Kindness in Therapy

There is no more plaintive complaint in mental healthcare than a want of kindness.[2] And there is no denying the fact that greater 'kindness' enhances all our therapeutic relationships. Mental healthcare literature confirms this fact. Kindness promotes healing

---

[2] J. Ballatt and P. Campling, *Intelligent Kindness: Reforming the Culture of Healthcare*, RCPsych Publications, 2007.

and so it fosters the recovery of a well-lived life. A more 'intelligent kindness' is required to reform our healthcare culture. No one thinks this is going to be easy. Healthcare is demanding work. Those of us working in healthcare are real people, and we are not angels. Intelligent kindness is not a sham. It cannot be a mask for the many unconscious and unresolved conflicts that exist within our services, and between our staff and our patients. The Francis Report into the calamitous NHS Mid-Staffordshire Hospital made this point very clearly. Staff are likely to experience a lack of kindness in services which are manifestly unkind to their patients.

A more 'intelligent kindness' could mobilize human kinship across services and multidisciplinary teams in the interests of recovery and the restoration of wellness. As Bertrand Russell said, 'The only thing that will redeem mankind is cooperation.' Individuals in mental distress are far more likely to recover when shown such kindness, and those caring for them are far more likely to survive as carers if they experience this kindness themselves.

Inevitably, the industrialization of our healthcare system and its fragmentation (particularly in mental healthcare) have not helped to foster a culture of kinship or kindness. Ultimately this cultural loss represents a crisis of clinical leadership. The former Deputy Chief of the NHS Services in England and Wales, the late Professor Aidan Halligan, certainly came to this view. His team conducted a large number of investigations into some of the most infamous scandals in the NHS, most notably the Harold Shipman scandal, in which an apparently avuncular and outwardly kindly GP turned out to be a sadistic serial killer in disguise. No one stopped Dr Shipman until it was too late. Perhaps no one could. In the future effective clinical leadership is needed to restore trust and kindness in our health services and the actions required cannot be too technological or obscure. As Professor Halligan used to say, 'It's about doing the right thing on a difficult day.' Actually that's quite a challenge.

Afterword: Mindful Recovery

MINDFULNESS CLEARLY PLAYS AN important part in the recovery of a life well lived. In a general sense mindfulness represents a renewed consciousness, one that is truly lived in the present and in a non-judgemental way. This mindfulness is a source of serenity and it surely helps us to be well. In this age of anxiety, we may need a more courageous consciousness, for ourselves and for each other, one that helps us to be truly present in a more connected and hopeful way.

Mindfulness is also useful in a more specific sense. The value of meditation has been demonstrated, and so mindfulness is a recognized form of 'therapy' in itself, but it is the benefit of mindfulness within modern therapy that has been the theme of this book. All these modern learning therapies include a portion of mindfulness practice. For example, Arthur in his experience of CFT and Patricia in her experience of DBT benefited from mindfulness as a part of their structured journey, moving them away from their self-reproach and their self-harm.

Mindfulness is not a panacea but it is especially useful as part of these focused therapies. Its incorporation speaks to the fact that modern therapy integrates wisdoms from a variety of sources in the interests of integrated human recovery.

Recovery is essentially about putting things back together again. Modern therapy brings together many ideas from many different sciences. By doing so, it helps people to find their integrity through the unity of health in mind and body. The childhood nursery rhyme 'Humpty Dumpty' tells us that 'all the king's horses and all the king's men couldn't put Humpty together again'. Experience of modern therapy tells me that in mental health this may not always be true.

Recovery is a legitimate expectation and it is a mindful one. Obviously it is a collaborative challenge, but the journey to a well-lived life through modern therapy is full of hope. In this journey we can rediscover peace and joy, love and laughter, and we can work again. We can expect to enjoy sport and music and art, and ultimately the fullness of human intimacy. With modern therapy we can rediscover all of this, mindfully, and in the context of everyday life.

For me, therapy is an invaluable tool for those on the route to wellness. The emphasis I have put on learning and on the therapeutic process is vitally important. This learning explains my enthusiasm for modern behavioural and cognitive therapies, and especially for some of the newer, more mindful variants described in this book.

There are only two ways of promoting wellness in my view. The first is by health promotion (education, or what we might call 'illness prevention') and the second is by investing in more effective mental healthcare.

Prevention is always better than cure. Illness prevention is the reason that we need to learn as early as possible how to promote resilience and become mindful and be well. Support for wellness should be the intention of all our personal and familial, political, spiritual and educational endeavours.

So the next step is to provide more effective mental healthcare. No economic, social or health service plan should advance without first addressing this question: What does this plan do for our mental health recovery and wellbeing? Our policies and our politics would surely change if we took this approach. We could address our health challenges and rebuild better routes to a well-lived life. All our lives would be better if we were to respond with an emphatic belief in one insight: there is no health without mental health.

So what happens if we too experience mental distress or difficulty? What then? In those times I believe it is essential that modern, effective and mindful mental healthcare is available in a timely manner. Other than prevention there is no better way of promoting wellness than therapy. It should not be too much to ask. Mental healthcare may be labour intensive, but few investments in health can deliver more for a society than improved mental healthcare.

I have not intended to put a limit to the number of therapies included in this plan. I have simply chosen a handful of which I have direct experience and about which there is some robust evidence base. The progress in mental healthcare is real, despite impressions to the contrary. Each of these therapies is progressive and effective and each delivers measurable results.

My advocacy for these treatments amplifies the voice of the real experts, those whose expertise has been earned by real experience of their mental distress: our patients. Through their goodwill and generosity, we have observed the therapeutic process and seen some of what it can achieve, first hand. Their journeys may not be over. They may be travelling towards a brighter future or even more challenging times, but they are now part of a process we call recovery. This is 'a life well lived'. It is fitting, therefore, that the last words of encouragement come from them: 'Live life well. Engage and you can be well.'

Further Reading

Ballatt, J. and P. Campling (2007) *Intelligent Kindness: Reforming the Culture of Healthcare.* RCPsych Publications.

Clare, A. (1976, 1980) *Psychiatry in Dissent: Controversial Issues in Thought and Practice.* Routledge.

Damasio, A. (2006) *Descartes' Error: Emotion, Reason and the Human Brain.* Vintage.

Daniel, B. and S. Wassell (2002) *Adolescence: Assessing and Promoting Resilience in Vulnerable Children* Vol. 3. Jessica Kingsley.

Dawkins, R. (2003) *A Devil's Chaplain: Reflections on Hope, Lies, Science, and Love.* Houghton Mifflin.

Fairburn, C. (2008) *Cognitive Behavior Therapy and Eating Disorders.* Guilford Press.

Freeman, H. (ed.) (2001) *A Century of Psychiatry.* Mosby Press.

Gilbert, P. (2010) *Compassion Focused Therapy.* Routledge.

Hayes, Steven C., Kirk D. Strosahl and Kelly G. Wilson (2012) *Acceptance and Commitment Therapy: The Process and Practice of Mindful Change* (2nd ed.). Guilford Press.

Jeffers, S. (2007) *Feel the Fear and Do It Anyway: How to Turn Your Fear and Indecision into Confidence and Action.* Vermilion.

Kelly, B. (2016) *Hearing Voices: A History of Irish Psychiatry.* Irish Academic Press.

Laing, R. D. (2010) *The Divided Self: An Existential Study in Sanity and Madness.* Penguin.

Linehan, M. (1993) *Cognitive-Behavioral Treatment of Borderline Personality Disorder.* Guilford Press.

McKay, M., J. C. Wood and J. Brantley (2007) *The Dialectical*

Behaviour Therapy Skills Workbook: Practical DBT Exercises for Learning Mindfulness, Interpersonal Effectiveness, Emotion Regulation and Distress Tolerance. New Harbinger Publications.

O'Mahony, G. and Lucey, J. V. (eds) (1998) *Understanding Psychiatric Treatment: Therapy for Serious Mental Health Disorder in Adults.* John Wiley and Sons.

Shore, David A. (2011) *The Trust Prescription for Healthcare: Building Your Reputation with Consumers.* Health Administration Press.

Shorter, E. (1997) *A History of Psychiatry: From the Era of the Asylum to the Age of Prozac.* John Wiley and Sons.

Stannard, R. (2000) *The God Experiment: Can Science Prove the Existence of God?* Hidden Spring.

Szasz, T. (1974) *The Myth of Mental Illness: Foundations of a Theory of Personal Conduct.* Harper and Row.

Williams, M. and D. Penman (2011) *Mindfulness: A Practical Guide to Finding Peace in a Frantic World* (foreword by Jon Kabat-Zinn, the originator of the mindfulness movement). Piatkus.

Wolfe, Brenda L. and Robert J. Meyers (2003) *Get Your Loved One Sober: Alternatives to Nagging, Pleading, and Threatening.* Hazeldon.

Acknowledgements

This book could not have been written without considerable help from many generous people, who were willing to share their experience in the hope that reading it might help someone other than themselves. I am particularly grateful to my friends Emma Farrell and Ronan Vaughan at Dogsear, Sheila Crowley at Curtis Brown, and Eoin McHugh and Brenda Kimber at Transworld Publishers.

The manuscript has been read many times by my colleagues and patients, and also by some friends with an expertise in mental healthcare. I owe a substantial debt to all these early readers for their encouragement and direction but particularly to Ms Charlotte Frorath, Ms Sarah Delaney, Ms Niamh Clarke, Dr Padraig Wright, Dr Anne-Marie O'Dwyer, Dr John Hillery, Dr Marie Naughton, Dr Clare Cullen, Dr Elaine Breslin, Dr Treasa O'Sullivan, Mr Seamus Brett, Ms Imelda McHugh and Mr Liam Hennessy. That said, if there are any errors or omissions in the text they are entirely my own. Please accept my apologies in advance.

I am also very grateful to all my colleagues at St Patrick's University Hospital in Dublin for their help during the preparation of the text, especially Ms Niamh O'Reilly (librarian), Ms Sarah Surgenor, Mr Tom Maher, Mr Paul Gilligan, Ms Anne Donnelly and Mr James Braddock.

Lastly, to my wife, Philippine, and our children, Mary, Hannah, Sarah, Michael and Philippa, my deepest gratitude goes to you for your patience and good humour during this and many other projects. I really hope you enjoy this book!

Index

depression (*cont.*)
  and self-esteem 168
  symptoms of 52–3
  what depression feels like 194
Descartes' Error 56
despair 66, 98, 216
detoxification 98, 100, 106
diagnosis of mental health 31–40
  differences in diagnosis 37
  treatment, determination by 35
Diagnostic and Statistical Manual
    (DSM) 33–4, 35, 39
Dialectical Behaviour Therapy (DBT)
    43–4, 70, 211–49
*Dialectical Behaviour Therapy Skills
    Workbook* 216
diaries
  behavioural diaries 172, 216
  childhood diaries 212, 219–20,
      222–4, 226, 231, 246
  cognitive diaries 55
  and Dialectical Behaviour Therapy
      (DBT) 213, 216
  eating diaries 79, 93
disappointments 169
disclosure, and stigma 19–21
dismissal of mental health problems
    253–4
distance, emotional 211–12
distraction activities 88
distraction plans 217
distress
  and Compassion Focused Therapy
      (CFT) 171
  distress call of the defensive system
      193
  and recovery 278
  tolerance of 192, 209, 216–17, 218,
      236
dopamine-based drive system 170–1
drugs 25
  and Acceptance and Commitment
      Therapy (ACT) 70, 97–130

eating disorders 40
  and control 75, 78
  and Enhanced Cognitive
      Behavioural Therapy for Eating
      Disorders (CBT-E) 70, 71–96
economy
  economic value of mental health 9–10
  economic wellbeing 10
  and resilient wellness 29
education 28–9
effectiveness 218
emotions
  accepting emotions 209
  emotional disregulation 213, 215
  emotional instability 215
  emotional regulation 216, 218, 237
  emotional resilience 26–9
  emotional wellness 9
  painful emotions 128, 211
empathy 42, 171, 192
emptiness, psychological 26
energy, loss of 33, 52–3
engagement
  and mindfulness 58
  re-engagement with life 22
  and recovery 69, 280, 287
  therapeutic engagement 40
  with therapy 1, 65, 95
Enhanced Cognitive Behavioural
    Therapy for Eating Disorders
    (CBT-E) 70, 71–96
environmental wellness 9
everyday stress 12
expansion, and Acceptance and
    Commitment Therapy (ACT) 99
exposure 43
  and Cognitive Behavioural Therapy
      (CBT) 55
  Exposure and Response Prevention
      (ERP) 44–5, 49

Fairburn, Professor Christopher 57, 72,
    93

296

panic disorders 43
the past 74
Pavlov, Ivan 43
perseverance 1
perspective taking 104
  and Acceptance and Commitment
    Therapy (ACT) 99
phobias 40
  and Behaviour Therapy (BT) 43, 44
  phobic anxiety 46
  phobic disorder 34
physical wellness 9
pie charts 86–7, 93
poetry 62
positive psychology 22–3
  positive values 28–9
post-traumatic stress disorder 40
  and alcohol abuse 134
  and depression 34
poverty, correlation with illness 10
protest 208
psych wars 49–50, 282
psychological medicine 16
  positive psychology 22–3
psychosis, Cognitive Behavioural
    Therapy (CBT) for 52
psychotherapy 61
  vs medicine 15–16
public awareness, increasing 18–19
purging 73, 75

rape 113, 115, 127
reality, imagined 212
reasoning 192
reassurance 170
recovery 69
  and acceptance 14–15
  capacity for recovery 21
  care plans 64
  and the good life 41–59
  and talking therapy 23–4
re-engagement with life 22
relaxation 217

resilience 14
  definition of 24–6
  emotional resilience 26–9
  six domains of resilience 28–9
response prevention 43
  Exposure and Response Prevention
    (ERP) 44–5, 49
rewards 170
road maps 155, 156–7, 164
rock bottom approach 132, 145, 157
Russell, Bertrand 284
Rutter, Sir Michael 27–8

sadness, persistent 33
safeness 170
schemas 54
schizophrenia 21, 212
  diagnoses 32, 33, 50
secrets 274, 280
security 28–9
self-acceptance 58, 271
self-blame 25–6, 34, 169
self-confidence, low 34
self-criticism 255
  behaviour diaries 172
  and being kind to yourself 180
  and Compassionate Focused
    Therapy (CFT) 170, 172, 193,
    209
  and Compassionate Mind Therapy
    (CMT) 171
  and harsh judgement in childhood
    168
self-destructive coping strategies 216
self-disclosure 20–1
self-esteem 168
self-harm 39, 227–8, 237, 243
  and coping strategies 216
  and Dialectical Behaviour Therapy
    (DBT) 238, 248
self-kindness 90
self-medication 127, 129
self-nurturing 168

ABOUT THE AUTHOR

Professor Jim Lucey is Clinical Professor of Psychiatry at Trinity College, University of Dublin, and Medical Director at St Patrick's University Hospital, Dublin. He has written numerous articles on the subject of mental health, having spent over thirty years working with individuals experiencing problems such as depression, anxiety, addiction, psychosis and suicidality. He is the author of two previous books, *Understanding Psychiatric Treatment* (co-edited with Dr G. O'Mahony) and the *Irish Times* bestseller *In My Room*. Jim lectures and conducts talks and seminars throughout Ireland, the UK and Europe and appears regularly on Irish radio and television to discuss issues of the mind and mental wellbeing. He lives in Dublin with his wife and family.